Neural Network Model: Applications and Implications

Series Editor

Theodore Wasserman Wasserman & Drucker PA, Boca Raton, FL, USA

More information about this series at http://www.springer.com/series/16167

Theodore Wasserman • Lori Wasserman

Motivation, Effort, and the Neural Network Model

Springer

Theodore Wasserman
Institution for Neurocognitive Learning Therapy
Wasserman & Drucker PA
Boca Raton, FL, USA

Lori Wasserman
Institution for Neurocognitive Learning Therapy
Wasserman & Drucker PA
Boca Raton, FL, USA

Neural Network Model: Applications and Implications
ISBN 978-3-030-58723-9 ISBN 978-3-030-58724-6 (eBook)
https://doi.org/10.1007/978-3-030-58724-6

This Springer imprint is published by the registered company Springer Nature Switzerland AG
The registered company address is: Gewerbestrasse 11, 6330 Cham, Switzerland

Preface

When we set out to write a book about motivation, we can honestly report that we were not entirely certain where we would wind up. That is in no small part due to the fact that Western sciences are often viewed as completely disparate. We were going to attempt to integrate research findings from a number of these seemingly disparate disciplines into a cogent, but new, comprehensive model. The fields of cognitive neuroscience, neurophysiology, clinical neuropsychology, and developmental neuroscience are all drawn upon to produce what we think is an integrated and conceptually intact whole that explains how the construct of motivation operates in the human brain.

This is not to say that we didn't have some conjectures about how it all might work, we did. We also had some ideas about what our findings might mean for the practice of clinical neuropsychology in particular and the treatment of mental health in general. We can now report to you that some of our ideas were right, and some of them needed modification. That is the way of science.

What is also clear at this point, is that some of our findings have potentially significant implications for important areas of neuropsychology and clinical psychology. Specifically, the implications of our work will impact issues such as effort testing in neuropsychology and improving motivation in clinical psychology. Our work will suggest some new ways of looking at these issues, and some new ways of assessing motivation in general. Candidly, the data we review suggest that some of the ways the field has been looking at these constructs may be in error. In other instances our work suggests that certain things the field has taken for granted may deserve a second look because, perhaps, we should have not been so certain about them in the first place. Finally, the work will suggest some entirely new directions, such as the creation of a completely new class of disorders of mental health based upon how the brain operates, rather than on the behavior it produces.

While we understand that some of our suggestions and conclusions will challenge some long-standing beliefs, it was not our intention to be contentious or to argue for one perspective or another. It was our intention to create a neural network based model of motivation and its related construct of effort and we went where the research took us. After reading our work, we hope you will agree with us about the necessity of endeavors such as this. We continue to believe that a neural network based reimagining of how neuropsychology views constructs such as motivation, effort, and mental health is fundamental for the health and advancement of our field.

After creating a network model, we attempted to look at some of the implications of that model for the field in general. We hope that you will consider our view of these implications. Our list is not exhaustive and we are sure that there are, and will be, many others. We also hope that we have provided you with enough data to generate your own ideas and form your own conclusions. We understand that there might be some disagreement about some of our implications, and we accept that as the process of science. Disagreement about the implications should in no way detract from the empirical validity of the model itself. We look forward to the continuing scientific dialogue.

Boca Raton, FL, USA

Theodore Wasserman
Lori Wasserman

Contents

Chapter 1
Introduction

Why would one write a book about motivation? Just as importantly, why would one invest hours in reading a book about motivation? As it turns out, asking ten people this question might well yield ten different responses, ranging from understanding motivation as it impacts self-improvement, to motivation as it impacts neuropsychology test results, to motivation in corporate leadership, to motivation as it impacts social psychology questions. And as it turns out, all of these diverse areas of interest would be spoken under the main umbrella of "motivation." In fact, a quick internet search of the term "motivation" yields well over one billion hits. A search through a national book store chain for books on "motivation" indicates over 5000 hits. A similar search on Google Scholar results in 3,970,000 hits. Surely all of these responses cannot be referring to the same construct. The answer is "maybe." When we look at the returned hits more closely, we see very long lists of concepts with one including instinct, drive, arousal, motive, self-empowerment, and self-improvement, another list of hits involving intrinsic vs. extrinsic motivation, followed by another seemingly never ending list which includes the external environment such as work or academics, and finally symptom validity and faking bad protocols in neuropsychological testing. Somehow, this vast collective of data, research and popular literature is all centered around a construct we call motivation. But, simply by observation of the vastness and diversity of the lists, we must conclude that motivation is a construct we only very poorly and widely define. What actually is this thing we call motivation? The dictionary describes motivation as a noun, and goes on to define it as an act or process, as in some students needing motivation, or as a condition, as in one who lacks motivation. Does then, this condition reside in our minds, or is it inferred based upon our body's movements and behavior, or by a lack thereof as we assess the process? How do we measure this thing called motivation? Is it by self-report? Is it by attainment of a goal, or by how much of the goal is attained, or is it by the amount of effort expended? And if it is by amount of effort expended, how do we gauge or quantify how much one was

T. Wasserman, L. Wasserman, *Motivation, Effort, and the Neural Network Model*, Neural Network Model: Applications and Implications,
https://doi.org/10.1007/978-3-030-58724-6_1

motivated to engage, and how much effort to expend? Did he in fact "try his best" or do we opine that he "is not really trying"? How do we make that judgment and how do we measure it? This is an important question as we do make these judgments every day when we assess student effort, test taking effort or workplace effort. Which brings us to the set of next questions: is what we are measuring a stable construct? Does it originate internally? And lastly, is motivation internally or externally governed?

For many people in the world of mental health, treatment, and research, addressing the mind–body problem is an active pursuit. It is under this umbrella that distinctly human constructs, such as emotions and drives are studied. The mind body problem essentially attempts to describe the relationship between the existential concept of mind and the physical reality of the body, in this case the brain. Is it one or the other that is the existential mind or the physical embodiment of the brain? Where does one start and one end? Is the whole greater than the physical sum of its parts? This relationship between mind and brain has always been the subject of dialogue and discourse, and to a large extent the answer, to this date, remains a mystery. The body's physical, spatially extended, and tangible reality seems to be radically different from the mental reality that can only be accessed through our own subjective consciousness (Oudenhove & Cuypers, 2010). Principally, the mind is about mental processes, thought, and consciousness. The body is about the physical aspects of the neural architecture and how the brain is structured. The mind–body problem concerns itself with understanding how these two interact. Historically, they were considered different and separate things that either operated independently or interdependently. The mind was where emotions resided, and so when you spoke about anything related to how emotions affected the behavior of a human being, you were speaking about the mind. Mental processes often were conceptualized as distinct from physical processes and somehow independent of the physiology of the basis of their expression and operation. Some philosophers held that mental properties involving conscious experience had fundamental properties that were not governed by the laws of physics, while the body had fundamental properties that were entirely based on the operation of the human brain and its networked architecture.

This separation of things belonging to the mind and things belonging to the body, originating in the realm of philosophy, has extended into, and persisted since the beginning of the field of psychology, and by further extension, neuropsychology. It has allowed us to explore sophisticated mental constructs such as love, commitment, and greed. These constructs, cultivated and developed over many years, are firmly established in our psyche and in our science. However, they are accepted as reality even if the proof of their existence lies solely within the boundaries of our subjective mental experience. Many of these constructs are considered uniquely human and perhaps, existential. An attempt to better study these phenomena has led neuroscience in general, and neuropsychology and psychiatry in specific, to attempt to provide a body-based neural underpinning for the mental constructs. This has been difficult, and in some cases impossible to achieve because, oft times a construct, as currently conceptualized, is considered to be an independent phenomenon, thereby beyond or incompatible with the operation of the neural networks over which the information related to the construct must travel. To wit, how does one explain love?

There is increasing awareness that the mind–body distinction is a barrier to understanding the relationship of mind to body. This is because it has become increasingly clear that the dichotomy is a false one (Wasserman & Wasserman, 2016). With full respect from the current authors to the larger biological system, including sympathetic and parasympathetic nervous systems, whatever the monitoring and executive processes are that constitute the mind, they are conducted over the same neural circuitry as everything else that is learned and processed in the human brain (Bremner, 2002). The same rule therefore applies to motivation. Just as we are coming to understand that the brain is not modular, that we cannot talk about a process or by extension a construct in isolation, we need to address the reality that we cannot talk about motivation in isolation. This becomes clearer, or specifically the dilemma, becomes clearer, as we look at current definitions.

1.1 How Do We Determine the Definition of Motivation?

This book concerns itself with one mind-based construct that has profound implications for psychology and neuropsychology. That is the construct or idea of motivation. Motivation is a complex, mind-based construct that is used to describe, define, and/or account for purposeful, goal-directed aspects of human behavior. So how has understanding this amorphous construct been attempted? One way has been by trying to assess if this construct is internally or externally based. To this end, motivation has been categorized as being either extrinsic or intrinsic, depending upon the reinforcement aspects of the behavior or goal. That is, extrinsic or outcome-focused motivation drives actions aimed at reaching a desired end state, such as a particular academic or professional grade, level of income, etc. Intrinsic or process-focused motivation drives actions that, in and of themselves, constitute the desired end state (Kruglanski et al., 2018). An activity is defined as intrinsically motivated if it constitutes its own end (Laran & Janiszewski, 2010). In contrast to the extrinsic, when people's motivational focus is intrinsic, their motivation stems from internal rewards and increases as a function of the extent to which goal-related activities elicit positive feelings of enjoyment, interest, and satisfaction. Examples might include finishing a book while "reading for pleasure" or participating in volunteer work.

It is important to note that it is very difficult to get a clear definition of the construct of motivation independently from the temporal goal with which it is related. Research on motivation almost always occurs in relation to a specific goal. Subset areas invoking motivation include for example, motivation to learn, motivation to succeed, or motivation for self-improvement. In fact, it is very difficult to understand or assess the idea of motivation in the absence of a thing about which to be motivated. As a result, these subsets, all believed to be reflecting the construct of motivation, become almost independent of each other. For example, the motivation for self-improvement is represented by a dominant model that is hardly used at all when discussing academic-based motivation or motivation for financial success.

Compounding of the difficulties outlined above, specifically the idea of defining motivation as a discrete construct, occurs when one looks at the inverse relationship, that is, the effect of the goal defining the motive, or the fact that a given definition of a goal can imply vastly different assumptions about the source of motivation. For example, some theories define a goal as a desired end state, and examine the extrinsic or outcome-focused motivation to reach this end state or obtain external rewards (e.g., money, food, prizes). Based on this view, the end state or outcome of the action taken to reach the goal has a strong influence on motivation. This is often measured by the amount of effort (energy) expended by the individual to attain the goal. Conversely, there are models of motivation that define a goal as a desired state. These models imply that people are motivated to move in a certain direction, but not necessarily for the purpose of reaching an end state. For example, some people enjoy learning about things for the sake of learning, even if there is no direct or extrinsic benefit for the learning in question.

As a result, the field of motivation is confounded by a lack of clear definition of motivation, motivational constructs, and specification of their operation within larger theoretical frameworks. These ongoing problems have implications for interpretation of research results and applications to practice (Shunk, 2000).

1.2 How Do We Measure Motivation?

As a consequence of the definitional problems associated with the construct of motivation, the measurement of said motivation has been fraught with difficulties. Due to the fact that motivation is a mentalist, psychological construct that cannot be observed or recorded directly, studying it usually means that it is assessed by implication. Again, it is similar to the construct of reward. Most typically, investigators attempt to infer a measurement of motivation by way of observable cognitive (e.g., memory, perception), affective (e.g., subjective experience), behavioral (e.g., performance), and physiological (e.g., brain activation) responses as well as by using self-reports (Touré-Tillery & Fishbach, 2014). It should be stressed that motivation is almost always measured in relative terms. That is, it is compared to previous or subsequent levels of motivation or to motivation in a different goal state (e.g., salient vs. non-salient goal).

Given the fact that, as we have discussed, there are several different types of motivation defined in part by the type of goal being sought, an important consideration in determining the measurement of motivation, is understanding what type of motivation one is attempting to capture. They are not the same. The current authors have given consideration to the idea that some of this confusion could be addressed by incorporating multiple, and discerning words into our language to help delineate ostensibly different types of motivation. There is currently a distinction between outcome-focused motivation to complete a goal and the process-focused motivation to attend to elements related to the process of goal pursuit that has less emphasis on the outcome. For example, there is the intrinsic motivation that comes with achievement steps along the way to achieving a goal or objective, and the fact that some individuals are motivated by the pursuit of the goal itself (Ryan & Deci, 2000). Yet, we use the umbrella term of motivation to describe both. This is a significant complication in the world of neuropsychology and neuroscience as terms often drive research. One can see the corollary with the term ADHD and research findings. We now have three DSM categories with little distinction, and research which is often confounding secondary to a poorly defined term or diagnosis. With relation to theory development, the term has often been handled by describing mitigating variables. This will bring the current authors to discussions of curiosity, arousal, and reward later on, constructs implicit to motivation.

How we measure motivation is then, another issue. In some cases, particular measures of motivation may help distinguish between these different dimensions of motivation, whereas other measures may not. This has significant implications the implications of some of the findings of measures of motivation, and implications for clinical application: As Touré-Tillery and Fishbach point out, the measured speed at which a person works on a task can have several interpretations. Working slowly could mean (a) that the individual's motivation to complete the task is low (outcome-focused motivation); or (b) that their motivation to engage in the task is high such that they are enjoying the task (intrinsic motivation); or (c) that their motivation to "do it right" and use proper means is so intense that they are really focusing and applying themselves (means-focused motivation), or even (d) that they are tired (diminished physiological resources). In situations such as these interpretation is often based on context. As we will see later, this issue becomes significant and contentious when talking about the idea of motivation in forensic situations or motivation to perform on psychological tests. When we talk about motivation in these contexts, we will have to discuss the concept of effort and its relationship to motivation. We will see how these two concepts are linked but remain dissociable.

1.3 Why this book?

What this book is not, is merely an exercise of physicalism whose core idea is that the human being, including the mind, is nothing but complex physical matter. When applied to the mind–brain problem, physicalism posits that the nature of mental properties (mental states or events, including beliefs, sensations, feeling, emotions) and of the subject having them, is purely physical (Oudenhove & Cuypers, 2010). This book is also not about dualism, a model in the mind-body discussion that contrasts with physicalism through the core idea that nonphysical substances and properties exist, besides physical substances and properties. Rather, what we hope to accomplish in writing this book is to provide the reader with a relevant and current, unifying and neuroscience-based model as it applies to the practice of psychology. The current authors have previously provided unifying models which are network based, and incorporate biological, physiological, developmental, and life course factors. This undertaking is similarly an attempt to provide a unifying model of motivation, which has at its core, a network-based scheme that identifies the neural network based properties of goal seeking behavior (motivation) within a developmental/life course perspective. The implications of such a model are profound when applied to the clinical practice of psychology and neuropsychology.

In part, this work attempts to operationalize the set of five principles put forth by Kandel (1998) and others. Principle 1 is most closely aligned with the ensuing discussion.

> All mental processes, even the most complex psychological processes, derive from operations of the brain. The central tenet of this view is that what we commonly call mind, is a range of functions carried out by the brain. The actions of the brain underlie not only relatively simple motor behaviors, such as walking and eating, but all of the complex cognitive actions, conscious and unconscious, that we associate with specifically human behavior, such as thinking, speaking, and creating works of literature, music, and art. As a corollary, behavioral disorders that characterize psychiatric illness are disturbances of brain function, even in those cases where the causes of the disturbances are clearly environmental in origin (Kandel, 1998).

We have made this point as regards issues of mental health (Wasserman & Wasserman, 2016, 2017). This work attempts a fusion of cognitive neuroscience and the construct of motivation by describing how the construct is put together and expressed by the various network functions and properties of the human brain. In addition, we will point out where this new model leads to implications that are not consistent with current practices and paradigms. When these inconsistencies are identified, we provide suggestions concerning how these practices may need to be amended going forward.

References

Bremner, D. (2002). *Does stress damage the brain*. New York: W.W. Norton.

Kandel, E. R. (1998). A new intellectual framework for psychiatry. *American Journal of Psychiatry, 155*, 457–469.

Kruglanski, A., Fishbach, A., Woolley, K., Bélanger, J., Chernikova, M., Molinario, E., & Pierro, A. (2018). A structural model of intrinsic motivation: On the psychology of means-ends fusion. *Psychological Review, 125*(2), 165–182. https://doi.org/10.1037/rev0000095.

Laran, J., & Janiszewski, C. (2010). Work or fun? How task construal and completion influence regulatory behavior. *Journal of Consumer Research, 37*(6), 967–983.

Oudenhove, L., & Cuypers, S. (2010). The philosophical "mind-body problem" and its relevance for the relationship between psychiatry and the neurosciences. *Perspectives in Biology and Medicine, 53*(4), 545–557.

Ryan, R. M., & Deci, E. L. (2000). Self-determination theory and the facilitation of intrinsic motivation, social development, and well-being. *American Psychologist, 55*, 68–78.

Shunk, D. (2000). Coming to terms with motivation constructs. *Contemporary Educational Psychology, 25*, 116–119. https://doi.org/10.1006/ceps.1999.1018.

Touré-Tillery, M., & Fishbach, A. (2014). How to measure motivation. *A guide for the experimental social psychologist social and personality psychology compass, 8*(7), 328–341. https://doi.org/10.1111/spc3.12110.

Wasserman, T., & Wasserman, L. D. (2016). *Depathologizing psychopathology: The neuroscience of mental illness and its treatment*. Springer International Publishing. https://doi.org/10.1007/978-3-319-30910-1.

Wasserman, T., & Wasserman, L. D. (2017). *Neurocognitive learning therapy: theory and practice*. Cham: Springer International Publishing : Imprint: Springer.

Chapter 2
Traditional Models of Motivation

As this book is about neural network models of motivation, incorporating a developmental perspective, and a unifying model across disciplines, it is appropriate to provide a review of the major historical models of motivation for perspective. It is fair to say that psychologists and others have been talking about motivation for more than 100 years.

Psychologists who study motivation look at.

- What the individual is doing, or the choice of behavior,
- How long it takes before an individual initiates the activity, or the latency of behavior,
- How hard the person actually works at the activity, or the intensity of behavior,
- How long the individual remains at the activity, or the persistence of behavior, and
- What the individual is thinking and feeling during or after the activity, or the cognitions and emotional reactions that accompany or follow the behavior.

Consistent across the above is a focus on a specific temporal sequence leading to an achievement. Also consistent with the above is the study of the assumed initiating factor, being what we have traditionally coined motivation. There are many ways that the construct has been described, and many models put forward that purport to show how it operates. The definitions of motivation usually relate to the process, wherein goal-directed activities are both initiated and sustained. This is quite different from the study of achievement itself (Graham & Weiner, 2012) or goal attainment, which can be quantified and measured both across time and skill sets. In this way, the study of motivation is more akin to a post hoc measure of getting ready to learn, as opposed to assessing the magnitude of the learning itself.

Historically speaking, the question of behavior and intent can traced back to theology, and the ideas of free will vs. divine determinism. Much discourse has been

T. Wasserman, L. Wasserman, *Motivation, Effort, and the Neural Network Model*, Neural Network Model: Applications and Implications,
https://doi.org/10.1007/978-3-030-58724-6_2

devoted to the concept of human will and action with the question of it being fixed and divinely determined, or subject to free will and an association with the divine. The concept of 'moral motivation' dates back to Plato. This theological fusion later gave way to the concepts of free will and personally determined motivation as noted by philosophers such as Sartre.

As science became more acceptable, the nature of explaining human behavior changed. This gave rise to theories and models of content, or need-driven theories of motivation vs. process of cognitive theories of motivation based upon conscious human decision. The later shift from more philosophical to scientific efforts, content driven, may be exemplified by the shift from 'moral' motivation to the concepts of instincts, drives, and needs. Instinct motivation, behaviors consistent across species and without conscious thought, addressed a purely biologically driven explanation. The shift then moved to the attempts to describe the nature of drives and needs, perhaps best exemplified by Maslow (1943) which is discussed further below. Maslow, in what was revolutionary for his time, attempted to tie the continuum of biological needs with higher order pursuits, or self-actualization. This concept might now be considered self-determination.

There are several major models decidedly known as self-determination models for motivation. While each of these models has a somewhat different major focus, they are all recognizing the complexity of the construct, and attempting to deconstruct it into discrete, but associated factors. For example, self-determination theory proposes that maximum performance results from actions motivated by intrinsic interests or by extrinsic values that have become integrated and internalized. In these self-determination models, motivation serves to satisfy basic psychosocial needs such as autonomy and competence, and relatedness promotes such motivation (Cook & Artino, 2016).

In expectancy–value theory, motivation is a function of the anticipation of success in obtaining the desired goal in relation to the perceived value of the goal. Motivation is greatest when both expectancy of success and goal value are high, but disappears when one of these factors equals zero.

Attribution theory focuses on the causal attributions learners create to explain the results of an activity. Attribution theory classifies these attributions along several factors including their locus, stability, and controllability.

Social-cognitive theory stresses self-efficacy, the desire for self-improvement and value as the primary driver of motivated action. This model also identifies cues that influence future self-efficacy and support self-regulated learning.

Goal orientation theory posits that people tend to engage in tasks with the intent to master the content. This mastery is designed to do better than others or avoiding failure. Motivation psychology (Heckhausen & Heckhausen, 2018) is a more comprehensive model which speaks to the "whys" and "hows" of activities in pursuit of a particular goal. It understands motivation as a multifaceted concept, including goal-directed behavior (goal engagement and goal disengagement), for the purpose of control, and includes the volitional forces behind goal-directed behavior including thoughts, emotions, and skills. In order to understand goal-directed behavior, the model posits that it is necessary to explain intrinsic and extrinsic variables across the life span.

For us, the most interesting part of all of these models, and others, is the fact, with the exception of expectancy–value theory, the models all begin by assuming that motivation exists, and then progress forward to talk about how it works. None of the theories, until now, offers a discussion of how the construct of motivation would be created and maintained in the human brain. The closest that we can get to that level of conversation are the discussions of goal-directed behavior, but even then, a full discussion of how the brain drives goal seeking behavior has only very recently been available. We will review the above outlined models and others in the discussion below. We provide this review to provide a backdrop or frame of reference for our later discussion. As such, the reader interested in more detail about any of the models should begin with the original sources identified below. It is also important to know that motivational theories tend to vary by activity. Theories of academic motivation are often a bit different than theories of goal-directed behavior or theories of organizational improvement. We have tried to keep this discussion related to general themes or commonalities among these theories.

2.1 Maslow Hierarchy of Needs

Perhaps, the most widely recognized model of motivation is Maslow's Hierarchy of Needs (Maslow, 1943). Maslow hypothesized that individuals possessed an independent set of motivation systems that were unrelated to either rewards or unconscious desires, but more akin to instincts. Maslow believed that individuals are motivated to fulfill these certain inborn and predetermined sets of needs. These needs ranged from the most basic and largely biological, to more abstract drivers largely based on emotional and personality focused constructs. In his initial work, Maslow proposed that the more fundamental needs had to be obtained and satisfied before the higher order, more abstract needs were addressed. When one need was fulfilled, a person then seeks to fulfill the next one in the hierarchy, continuing in development until all needs were met. The original and most widespread version (Maslow, 1954) of Maslow's hierarchy of needs includes five motivational needs. These needs are represented as stages. At the lowest level of the pyramid are basic/primary needs, without which one cannot survive. These are termed deficiency needs and serve to motivate people when they are unmet in order to address the anxiety that would result from these needs not being met. Deficiency needs become stronger (more motivating) the longer the duration they are denied. Then come a middle set of needs (e.g., physiological, safety, love, and esteem) and finally, at the top, are growth needs (self-actualization). These needs are best viewed as support and development needs, the acquisition or satisfaction of which, make the person more complete and evolved. These needs are often represented as forming a pyramid.

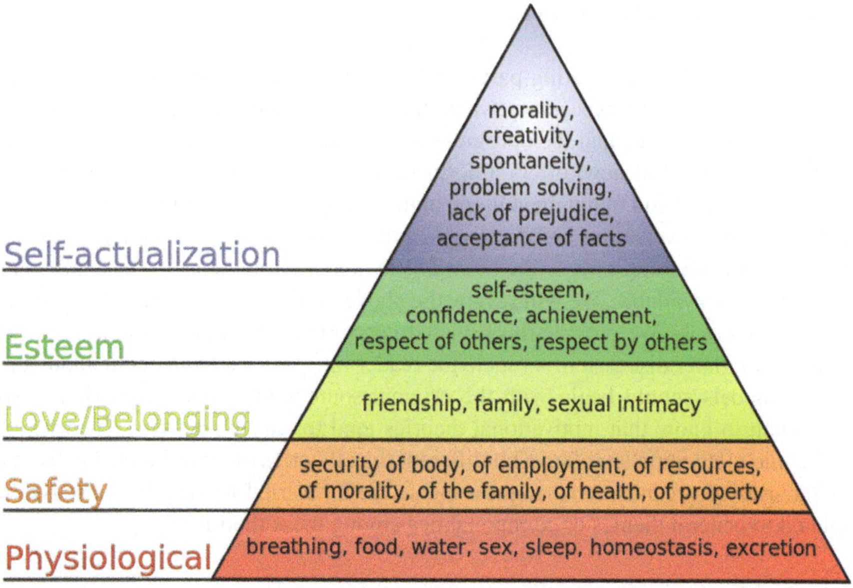

Maslow's Hierarchy of Needs. https://commons.wikimedia.org/wiki/User:J._Finkelstein

As originally conceived, an individual must satisfy lower level basic needs before progressing on to meet higher level growth needs. Once these needs have been reasonably satisfied, one may be able to reach the highest level called self-actualization. While every person is capable and has the inborn desire to move up the hierarchy toward self-actualization, development is often disrupted by failure to completely satisfy lower level needs. Life experiences including marriage, the birth of a child, divorce and successful employment cause people to fluctuate between levels of the hierarchy.

As can readily be seen, these needs represent basic physiological requirements, and also more abstract social and emotional constructs. They exist within the person. It could be argued that the higher order, more abstract needs, evolve from the more primary needs. Such an argument would be in line with developmental modeling and modeling based on the development of complex neural network-based goal seeking behaviors. Maslow did not make such arguments. He merely hypothesized that such needs exist and left it at that.

Despite remaining a very popular theory, there is little substantive research that supports the basic concepts of the theory. In particular, research has demonstrated that individuals can rapidly move between stages depending on the situation and circumstance. In fact, Maslow addressed this issue in his later work.

2.2 Self-Determination Theory

Other research has focused on self-determination and those factors which either enhance or undermine it. Self-determination theory attempts to incorporate biology, personality development, and social psychology issues. Self-determination theory points to three inherent growth stages (Ryan & Deci, 2000) or psychological needs. Those are competence, autonomy, and relatedness.

The conceptual foundation of self-determination theory (SDT) is based upon the premise that all people have natural, innate, and constructive tendencies to develop an increasingly elaborate sense of who they are, and their values (Deci & Ryan, 2008). In self-determination theory, human motivation and personality development concerns itself with people's inborn and constitutional tendencies for personal growth, and the impact of innate psychological needs on the development of the person. SDT proper focuses on the motivation behind the choices people make, exclusive of external influence and interference. Therefore, SDT focuses on the degree to which an individual's behavior is self-motivated and self-determined (Ryan & Deci, 2000). Intrinsic motivation refers to initiating an activity for its own sake because it is interesting and satisfying in and of itself. These drives are in opposition to doing an activity to obtain an external goal or reward (extrinsic motivation). The model describes different types of motivations based upon the degree to which they have been internalized. The process of internalization describes the active attempt to transform a previously extrinsic motive into personally endorsed, internal value. The model really concerns itself with already fully internalized drives.

The process of internalization involves the operation of three main needs that are inherent to all people in one way or the other. These needs are competence, relatedness, and autonomy. These needs are seen as universal necessities that are innate, not learned (instinctive), and seen in humanity across time, gender, and culture (Chirkov, Ryan, Kim, & Kaplan, 2003).

The three inherent drives or organizers of motivations are.

1. Competence, defined as the desire to seek and to control the outcome and experience mastery over the environment and oneself.
2. Relatedness, defined as the will to interact, be connected to, and experience caring for others.
3. Autonomy, defined as the desire to be causal agents of one's own life and act in harmony with one's integrated self.

What sets SDT apart from some other models is its willingness to consider what is motivating to a person at a specific time and circumstance as opposed to conceptualizing motivation as a unitary/fixed state-like concept. This consideration is significant to our future discussion of motivation in that neural network models of motivation will contain many state-like components when discussing motivated behavior. Traits are possible in neural models, but these traits represent response to similar stimuli rather than a universal tendency.

SDT does speculate that these innate motivational drives can be modified through interaction with the environment, particularly social contextual values, thereby making some of them stronger than others (Ryan & Deci, 2017). Social context is one way that this process occurs. As a result, there is room for the consideration of individual difference based upon a person's experience with the environment. This essentially replicates life course theory modeling which features prominently in discussion of neural network modeling (Wasserman & Wasserman, 2017). There are, therefore, large areas of overlap between neural network modeling and SDT in that understanding how neural networks develop and encode goal-directed behavior goes a long way toward understanding the process of internalization that figures so prominently in SDT theory.

2.3 Organismic Integration Theory

SDT makes distinctions between different types of motivation and the consequences of them. Ryan and Deci recognized that external stimuli can be motivating, that there are multiple types of external motivators, and that rewards are powerful drivers of behavior. They developed a sub-theory of SDT, called organismic integration theory (OIT), to account for and explain how these extrinsic variables impact and interface with the intrinsic variables identified in SDT (Deci & Ryan, 1985).

OIT describes four different types of extrinsic motivations. These are

1. Externally regulated behavior: This describes the impact of external reinforcement on human behavior. It describes behavior that is performed because of an external demand or possible reward.
2. Introjected regulation of behavior: This describes a person accepting regulations to their behavior, but not fully accepting said regulations as their own (Deci & Ryan, 1995). Examples of this type of motivation are what happen when a person seeks the approval of others, or considers the approval of other as essential to the development of their self-esteem. While the motivator here is internal, it is controlled by the external variable of 'other' approval. As a result of the causality of the behavior being external, the behavior is considered non-self-determined and, therefore, extrinsic.
3. Regulation through identification: This occurs when an originally external value or driver is internalized and considered by the individual as important in its own right.
4. Integrated regulation: This occurs when previously external regulations are fully internalized and integrated with an individual's belief and value system. As a result of their complete integration, integrated motivations share qualities with intrinsic motivation. They are however classified by Ryan and Deci as extrinsic because the goals that are trying to be achieved are for reasons extrinsic to the self, rather than the inherent enjoyment or interest in the task.

2.4 Expectancy–Value Theory

Expectancy–value theories will feature heavily in our network discussion of motivation. As a result, we will discuss them in general here, and in more detail later. Expectancy–value theory holds that the strength of a tendency to act in a certain way depends upon the strength of an expectation that the act will be followed by a given outcome, and on the degree of attractiveness of that outcome to the individual (Parijat & Bagga, 2014).

Overall, expectancy–value theories identify two key independent factors that influence behavior. The first of these is the degree to which people believe they will be successful, and obtain their goal, if they try. This is often termed expectancy of success. The second is the degree to which people perceive that there is a personal importance, value or intrinsic interest in doing the task. This is often termed task value.

Expectancy of success represents a future-oriented conviction that one can accomplish the anticipated task. If a person does not believe that they will be successful in accomplishing a task, they are unlikely to begin. Beliefs related to competence can be both general (e.g., global self-concept) and specific (judgments of ability to learn a specific skill or topic). Expectancy of success is shaped by motivational beliefs that fall into three broad categories: goals, self-concept and task difficulty. Goals refer to specific short- and long-term learning or mastery objectives. Self-concept refers to general impressions concerning the person's capacity in the task domain in question (Wigfield & Eccles, 2000). Task difficulty is of course, just that, as perceived by the observer.

As we have indicated, personal motivation requires more than just a belief that a person can be successful in obtaining the desired goal. In order to be selected, the goal has to have some personal value. Usually, the goal that is selected as the most motivating is the goal that will be pursued, as it is the goal that is valued the most. Like expectancy of success, task value or valence is relative, and idiosyncratic, to the person. There is no system of absolute value attributed to any goal or objective. For example, some people would give anything to secure World Series baseball tickets, while for others who don't follow baseball, these tickets are almost valueless.

Research has identified a number of factors as contributing to task value (Heckhausen & Heckhausen, 2018; Wigfield & Eccles, 2000):

1. A given topic might be particularly interesting or enjoyable. This is termed interest or intrinsic value.
2. Learning or mastering a skill or subject is often perceived as necessary and important for practical reasons, or a necessary step toward a future goal. This is termed utility or extrinsic value.
3. Successfully learning or mastering a skill or subject might hold personal importance in its own right, or as a statement of the individual's self-concept. This is termed importance or attainment value.
4. Focusing time and energy on one task means that other tasks are neglected. This is often termed opportunity cost or goal engagement cost (Heckhausen &

Heckhausen, 2018). The term goal disengagement refers to those goals not chosen for action. Other costs and potential negative consequences include anxiety, effort, and the possibility of failure.

5. The degree to which the attainment of the goal outcome permits the person to control their environment. The greater the control provided, the greater the value of the target goal.

There are of course things that shape and contribute to the idiosyncratic determination of relative value. Value is hypothesized to be shaped by motivational belief: emotionally based memories, emotions that are based on prior experiences. Positive experiences develop perceived value; unfavorable experiences lessen it. Expectancy–value theory plays an integral part in understanding how motivation develops within the context of a neural network model. As such we will have more to say on that subject later.

2.5 Attribution Theory

Attribution theory (Weiner, 2000) is a theory that tries to explain why individual people react differently to a specific experience. Attribution theory posits that different responses arise from differences in the perceived cause of the initial outcome, or simply put, how we explain it. A major emphasis in this model is the difference between attributions based on internal factors such as motivation and drive, and external factors such as luck or family connections. The attribution of success or failure in mastering a new skill, or being successful in an endeavor, can be attributed by the person to a number of factors such as personal effort, innate ability, other people (e.g., the teacher) or luck. While these actions are often subconscious, they nevertheless influence future activities. Failure attributed to lack of ability might suppress future effort, while failure attributed to poor training or bad luck might encourage the motivation to try again.

Integrating with a value expectancy model, attributions would be construed to directly influence expectancy of future success, and indirectly influence perceived value as mediated by the individual's emotional response to success or failure.

Attribution theory proposes that people have a default goal of understanding and mastering both themselves and the environment. People develop cause–effect models for the events in their lives. The process of attribution begins with an event, such as mastering a skill or the successful outcome of an event. Whether the outcome is positive or negative, the learner makes attributions regarding how the event happened and what caused the result. The attributions can be positive or negative, internal or external, or stable and unstable. For example, winning a hand of poker can be attributed to a well-developed and stable skill that permitted understanding of the odds of each hand developing, or might on the other hand, be attributed to luck. Internal, positive and stable attributions would lead hypothetically, to increased motivation. In this model attributions do not directly motivate behavior. Rather, they are interpreted or reframed into psychologically meaningful (actionable) responses that may drive future behavior (Cook & Artino, 2016).

As in expectancy–value theory, attributions are linked to motivation through the constructs of expectancy of success and task value (Weiner, 2000). Expectancy of success is directly influenced by perceived causes that are related to the stability dimension. If conditions (the presence or absence of causes) are expected to remain the same, then the outcome(s) experienced in the past will be more likely to occur in the future. If the causal conditions are perceived as likely to change, then there is likely to be uncertainty about subsequent outcomes. Success and certainty lead to motivate behavior.

2.6 Social-Cognitive Theory

Social-cognitive theory can alternately be described as a theory of learning as opposed to a theory of motivation. Specifically, social-cognitive theory posits that people use cognition to mediate between rewards and actions. Cognition (thinking, internalized thoughts) determines how people interpret their environment and self-regulate their thoughts, feelings, and actions. This is an active process of regulating behavior and manipulating the environment in pursuit of personal goals. This set of actions is fundamental to the functioning of a motivated person. Whether or not people actually choose to pursue their goals depends on beliefs about their own capabilities, values, and interests (Pajares, 2008), thereby affecting motivation.

The intersections of this model with both attribution theory and expectancy–value theory are evident. Specific to the social-cognitive model is the idea of self-efficacy. Self-efficacy is a belief about what a person can do and achieve rather than a personal judgment about one's physical or psychological attributes (Bandura, 1997). Looking at self-efficacy from an attributional perspective, self-efficacy is the belief that it was the person themselves, due to their skills, knowledge, and attributes that will cause the success of a particular action to happen.

Self-efficacy should not be confused with outcome expectation, which is the belief that a specific outcome will result from a given, specific action. The two constructs are however, typically, positively correlated due to the fact that self-efficacy beliefs help to determine the outcomes one expects; The greater my belief in my capabilities, the greater my belief in a particular outcome. It is nevertheless, the case that sometimes, self-efficacy and outcome expectations diverge. For example, a high-performing, highly efficacious college student may choose not to apply to the most elite law school because they believe that while their scores are high, they are not quite good enough for a particular school. They therefore anticipate a rejection. In this case, academic self-efficacy is generally high, but outcome expectations for a discrete event are low. Interestingly, research indicates that self-efficacy beliefs are usually better predictors of behavior than are outcome expectations (Zimmerman & Cleary, 2006).

2.7 Goal Orientation (Achievement Oriented) Models

Goal orientation models are very different from the models described above. Goal theory was originally a model used for investigating student learning. It intersects with self-regulation and cognitive motivational models. A goal orientation model fits well with self-regulated learning theory as a result of its assumption that in order for students to self-regulate learning, performance, and behavior, they must have some goal or standard or criterion against which to measure and compare their progress. Goal theory posits the idea that students have a general orientation to achievement tasks that can be described in terms of the three general orientations of mastery, extrinsic, and relative ability. If students adopt one orientation more than the others, then the setting of this general orientation or standard should be related to their use of various self-regulatory strategies that are inherent in the goal orientation strategy selected.

Goal orientation models appear to suggest that motivation is a goal specific, stable trait. Achievement Goal Orientation is a general motivation theory (Dweck & Leggett, 1988), which highlights the fact that the type of goal a person is working toward, has a significant impact on how intensely they pursue the goal. Intensity of pursuit is a stand in for motivation in this model. As indicated, goal orientation models have two and sometimes three, broad classes of goals (Pintrich, 1999). A mastery goal orientation refers to a concern with learning and mastering the task using self-set standards and self-improvement. This is an intrinsic set of goals. People with mastery goal orientations are willing to put forth a lot of effort to "master" a skill or concept. In general, people with a mastery goal orientation will work very hard, persist in the face of difficulty and frustration, will take risks and try things that they don't already know how to do.

Performance goal orientation is by contrast, frequently extrinsic in nature. It often includes for example, a focus on getting good grades and pleasing others (teachers, parents) as the main criterion for judging success. Finally, some models include a third class of goal orientation: A relative ability orientation refers to a concern with comparing one's ability or performance to others and trying to best them, to do better than them on the task.

Most interesting for a discussion of psychological practices, such as the ongoing debate about effort testing, these models suggest that these goal orientations are relatively stable and enduring over time. For example, people with performance goal orientations have an often subconscious self-theory that intelligence or ability is a stable and fixed trait. For individuals with this perspective, people are often grouped into one discrete group of intelligence: either smart or not. As these performance goals are considered stable traits that cannot be changed, people are concerned about looking and feeling like they have enough of the particular skill or ability in question. This requires that they perform well and can therefore be motivating (Cook & Artino, 2016). In the alternative, people with this orientation who believe that they are not very smart are frequently unmotivated in academic settings, believing that there is nothing they can do to alter the outcome of events.

2.8 Unified Theories of Motivation

As should now be readily apparent, there are numerous theories that attempt to describe how motivation works. Each of these theories has a significant number of proprietary constructs. There have been attempts to integrate these disparate models into a coherent whole. For example, Dweck (2017) proposed a theory that attempted to integrate the constructs of motivation, personality, and development within one framework, using a common set of principles and mechanisms. The theory is based on a foundation that is comprised of basic needs, highly similar to those proposed by Maslow. These needs are those that, at the beginning, represent the necessity of survival. The actions people take, and the emotions and cognitions related to the actions, build into increasingly complex mental representations of these experiences (beliefs, representations of emotions, and representations of action tendencies). These internalized mental representations, comprised of needs, goals, success calculations, and value expectancies serve as the basis of both motivation and personality. The model also provides a new perspective on development, particularly on the forces that propel development and the highly integrated roles of nature and nurture. These integrative attempts are in the early stages of development. In general, there has yet to be a widely accepted broad, integrated theory of motivation. As a result any particular theory necessarily deals with only a subset of motivational factors (Steel & Konig 2006).

From our review, it appears that contemporary theories of motivation share at least four areas of belief. These are competence (the likelihood of success) beliefs, value beliefs, attribution, and social-cognitive interpretations. These appear to represent foundational principles that underpin a nuanced and integrative understanding of the role of the individual theories in a more global understanding of the construct. Major definitional and conceptual differences remain between the various models (Cook & Artino, 2016). It is not the intention of this book to integrate these models and settle these differences on a construct/semantic based level. It is the purpose of this book to underlie these constructs with a thorough understanding of how the construct of motivation, particularly these four common themes, might be created and composed by the brain. For example, how does the brain calculate or understand a construct like "the likelihood of success."

As we will see, each of the models outlined above make a valuable and creative contribution to the understanding of what motivation is. This is especially true when the model is filtered through the lens of neural network/ probabilistic reward valuation modeling. As we found when discussing the relative contribution of clinical models to an understanding of mental health (Wasserman & Wasserman, 2017), with this framework in place it becomes possible to create a truly integrative and understandable model of motivation.

References

Bandura, A. (1997). *Self-efficacy: The exercise of control*. New York: W.H. Freeman.

Chirkov, V., Ryan, R. M., Kim, Y., & Kaplan, U. (2003). Differentiating autonomy from individualism and independence: A self-determination perspective on internalisation of cultural orientations, gender and well being. *Journal of Personality and Social Psychology, 84(1)*, 97–110. https://doi.org/10.1037/0022-3514.84.1.97.

Cook, D., & Artino, A., Jr. (2016). Motivation to learn: An overview of contemporary. *Medical Education, 50*, 997–1014. https://doi.org/10.1111/medu.13074. The Cross Cutting Edge. Retrieved from https://onlinelibrary.wiley.com/doi/pdf/10.1111/medu.13074.

Deci, E. L., & Ryan, R. M. (1985). *Intrinsic motivation and self-determination in human behaviour*. New York: Plenum.

Deci, E. L., & Ryan, R. M. (1995). Human autonomy: The basis for true self-esteem. In M. Kemis (Ed.), *Efficacy, agency, and self-esteem* (pp. 31–49). New York: Plenum.

Deci, E. L., & Ryan, R. M. (2008). Self-determination theory: A macrotheory of human motivation, development, and health. *Canadian Psychology/Psychologie Canadienne, 49*(3), 182–185.

Dweck, C. (2017). From needs to goals and representations: Foundations for a unified theory of motivation, personality, and development. *Psychological Review, 124*(6), 689–719.

Dweck, C., & Leggett, E. (1988). A social-cognitive approach to motivation and personality. *Psychological Review, 95*, 256–273.

Graham, S., & Weiner, B. (2012). Motivation: Past, present, and future. In K. Harris, S. Graham, T. Urdan, C. McCormick, G. Sinatra, & J. Sweller (Eds.), *APA educational psychology handbook, Vol. 1. Theories, constructs, and critical issues* (pp. 367–397). Washington, DC: American Psychological Association. https://doi.org/10.1037/13273-013.

Heckhausen, J., & Heckhausen, H. (2018). *Motivation and action: Introduction and overview*. Cambridge: Cambridge Universtiy Press.

Maslow, A. H. (1943). A theory of human motivation. *Psychological Review, 50*(4), 370–396.

Maslow, A. H. (1954). *Motivation and personality*. New York: Harper and Row.

Pajares, F. (2008). Motivational role of self-efficacy beliefs in selfregulated learning. In D. Schunk & B. Zimmerman (Eds.), *Motivation and self-regulated learning: Theory, research, and application* (pp. 111–139). New York: Routledge.

Parijat, P., & Bagga, S. (2014). Victor Vroom's expectancy theory of motivation – An evaluation. *International Research Journal of Business Management, VII*(9), 1–8.

Pintrich, P. (1999). The role of motivation in promoting and sustaining self-regulated learning. *International Journal of Educational Research, 31*, 459–470.

Ryan, R., & Deci, E. (2017). *Self determination theory : Basic psychological needs in motivation and wellness*. New York: The Guilford Press.

Ryan, R. M., & Deci, E. L. (2000). Self-determination theory and the facilitation of intrinsic motivation, social development, and well-being. *American Psychologist, 55*, 68–78.

Steel, P., & Konig, C. (2006). Intergating theories of motivation. *Academy of Management Review, 31*(4), 889–913.

Wasserman, T., & Wasserman, L. (2017). *Neurocognitive learning therapy: Theory and practice*. New York: Springer.

Weiner, B. (2000). Intrapersonal and interpersonal theories of motivation from an attributional perspective. *Educational Psychological Review, 12*(1), 1–14.

Wigfield, A., & Eccles, J. (2000). Expectancy-value theory of achievement motivation. *Contemporary Educational Psychology, 25*, 68–81. https://doi.org/10.1006/ceps.1999.1015.

Zimmerman, B., & Cleary, T. (2006). Adolescents' development of personal agency: The role of self-efficacy beliefs and self-regulatory skill. In F. Pajares & T. Urdan (Eds.), *Self efficacy beliefs of adolescents* (pp. 45–70). Greenwich, CT: Information Age Publishing.

Chapter 3
The Development of Motivation

How plausible is it to think about motivation as something that you are born with. How many times have we heard someone who we describe as a "high achiever" described as having been "born that way"? Yet, on the other hand, how many of us have described the behavior of new born infants as motivated? When we describe the behavior of infants we do say things like driven, instinctual, or purposeful. We usually do not describe the infant's behaviors as motivated. Yet, it is quite probable that it is from those inborn, motor, cerebellar-driven behaviors, that motivation is developed. Furthermore, it is also not likely that motivation is something that just appears, fully articulated at some point in time. Motivation, like most other complex human behaviors, develops over time. At some as yet indeterminate point, the term drive is replaced with the term motivation (Deci & Moller, 2005) and, from that point, the proposition that all behavior is motivated is amply substantiated and generally accepted. This is commonly taken to mean that every strand of behavior can be traced to a particular drive or combination of drives. If we are going to have a model that understands how motivation is produced by an integrated neural network system, we need to have an idea of how that system develops the capability to produce the complex behavior that characterizes the construct of motivation.

We will base our model for the development of motivation on a number of sources but, in addition to our own work (Wasserman & Waserman, 2016), three sources stand out and will be used extensively. The first is a discussion of the developmental prospective regarding the development of cognition described in the work of Piaget (Piaget & Inhelder, 1972). The second is the role of movement and related behavior in the development of complex human functioning (Koziol & Budding, 2009; Koziol, Budding, & Chidekel, 2012). The third is a sociological perspective on the role of conflict, arousal and curiosity in the development of human higher order thought (Berlyne, 1960). Berlyne focuses on three general areas of study in the development of his model: (1) Internal Predisposing Factors, (2) The Nature of Reward (reinforcement) and, (3) Biological Utility. The goal for the current authors

T. Wasserman, L. Wasserman, *Motivation, Effort, and the Neural Network Model*, Neural Network Model: Applications and Implications,
https://doi.org/10.1007/978-3-030-58724-6_3

is again, to find the common cores and etiologies from a neuropsychological perspective. The current chapter explores the origins of the integration of stimuli, reflexive behaviors and associative learning, including reward. We will then explore more planned and directed behavior. We will posit that curiosity in particular, forms the basis for the development of complex human constructs in general, and motivation in particular.

Throughout this book we will look at these areas from a neural network perspective and talk about inborn and constitutionally predisposing factors, the reward recognition network and probabilistic reward calculations, and factors contributing to probabilistic reward calculation such as ease of obtaining, or the effort involved, in obtaining a particular goal or reward.

3.1 From Piaget to a Vertical Brain Model: Cortical and Subcortical Involvement in Child Development and the Etiology of Motivation

While much of what Piaget is known for resides in later stages, there had to be an accounting of the early stages of development of the human infant. Toward this end, Piaget talked about the initial stage known as the sensorimotor stage. This stage begins at birth and extends to the acquisition of language with the first substage consisting of reflexive behaviors. For our purposes, let us consider a reflex such as a rooting response, a response absolutely necessary for survival. During this stage, "infants develop an understanding of the world through trial and error using their senses and actions (i.e., motor movements)" (McLeod, 2009). Again, for example, notable in the newborn's expression of rooting behavior through head turning and mouth movements. Even at this early a point in life, it is clear that the neonate will turn toward the stimulus in an effort to locate the nipple for feeding. Even at this rudimentary stage, the child will attend to external sensory information, perhaps maternal smell and or having its cheek stimulated, and self-correct its locating skills in a necessary effort to obtain life sustaining sustenance. It is the basis of eons of evolutionary protection for survival. The infants will go on to build their base of knowledge and understanding of the world by coordinating their experiences obtained through e.g., vision and hearing, and from physical interactions with objects, through rudimentary reflexive behaviors such as sucking and grasping. As they mature through this stage, they progress from reflexive, instinctual behaviors toward the beginning of purposeful intent, for example, from exploration to search behavior, which better develops toward the end of this sensorimotor stage.

What Piaget described on a behavioral or biological level, Koziol described on a neural network level. The work of Koziol and Budding (2009) is based on the idea that "cognitive and affective regulations comprise extensions of motor control systems" (p. 14). With a vertical brain perspective, he highlighted the role of subcortical structures, including the basal ganglia on the development of all human cognition.

The basal ganglia, bilaterally represented gray matter, consists of four structures, notably the striatum, the pallidum, the substantia nigra which resides in the midbrain and the subthalamic nucleus. The basal ganglia are involved in a variety of tasks including motor skills learning, perceptual motor learning, cognitive skill learning, category learning, error analysis, and sequence learning. The basal ganglia operate based upon reward-driven associative learning. It also is concerned with intention, that is, how to gate our attention and select a particular response. This works together with the cerebellum, whose role in making error corrections, plays a pivotal role in the development of valuations, which we might all agree, lies at the core of motivated behavior.

The historical view of the basal ganglia as limited to involvement with motor behavior has been largely disproven in recent years (Middleton, 2000). Middleton et al. point to three lines of evidence; the first is the result of anatomical studies which clearly indicate the involvement of the basal ganglia in neural pathways with cognitive areas of the cerebral cortex. That is, the basal ganglia participate in a cerebellar-basal ganglia, cortical loop. Next is the activity of neurons within the basal ganglia which are more related to cognitive or sensory operations than they are to motor function. Lastly, in some cases, lesions in the basal ganglia cause primarily cognitive or sensory disturbances, while gross motor function remains intact.

We concern ourselves for the moment with the striatum, the single largest structure and primary region of all sensory input into the basal ganglia. The striatum consists of the dorsal striatum, which includes the caudate and the putamen, and ventral striatum. The latter contains the nucleus accumbens. The nucleus accumbens is, phylogenically speaking, an old structure, and of import, a reward center, with the shell concerned with consummatory reward. It projects to the ventral pallidum, an area associated with movement. This supports the idea that movement and motivation are tied both from an evolutionary standpoint and in terms of residual or current functioning (Aboitz, 2003). To emphasize the point, reward is calculated early on with the development of movement, implying the beginning of rewarded intent.

The striatum resides in a loop that connects the cortex to the thalamus, and then back to cortex. Projections into the striatum from the cortex are excitatory and are active only when required. This makes sense as it allows for the conservation of energy. One region of the cortex may project to more than area in the striatum, and one striatal zone may have projections from more than one cortical area. That is, the striatum receives information from cortical areas which include sensorimotor, associative and limbic areas. This makes sense as the neural networks of the brain have to interface for effective attention, evaluation, learning, and eventually response. The striatum receives dopamine-based connections from the midbrain. Again, we point out that this becomes important as we recall that the basal ganglia is involved with reward-driven associative learning. The striatum has been found to be extremely sensitive to environmental context. It receives sensory information about object identification, object location, and about internal states as well, which includes the goals and purpose of the organism as a whole (Saint-Cyr, 2003). Here again, we highlight the emerging coordination of input, learning and reward.

Koziol and Budding (2009) go on to highlight that the basal ganglia structure, as noted above, is phylogenetically very old, and was preserved and improved because of its value. Specifically, later on in development these regions support the integration of motivation with sensory input and motor input. Coupled with the importance of the cerebellum, their thesis is that the brain evolved for the control of action, rather than for the development of cognition. They proposed a definition and model of executive function whose development was based on continuous sensorimotor interaction with the environment. They hypothesized that procedural (skill) learning contributed to, and was the basis of, the acquisition of declarative (semantic) knowledge (Koziol et al., 2012).

Lastly, with respect to neural pathway impact on the developing system, it is important to note that processing requires energy. The human brain is designed to assess while, at the same time, conserve energy. In its assessment role, two types of processing have been addressed. These are stimulus-based processing and higher-order control processing categories (Koziol & Budding, 2009). Stimulus-based processing includes reflexes, and later on, habits and learned skills and procedures. This mode of responding employs behaviors utilized on a routine basis, allowing fast responsivity to assure survival and conservation of energy. The higher order processing comes online for novel situations requiring problem solving. This category of processing is time and energy consuming, but flexible, determining whether any given behavioral response will work or need to be modified. Each system has its advantages, and drawbacks. Evolution, or nature, decided to incorporate both systems into what is known as the frontostriatal system, a system allowing for the engagement of network loops as required by the task at hand. This allows for allows for conservation of energy for tasks which are becoming automatic, or have attained automaticity, while engaging and utilizing greater energy when encountering novel stimuli.

Development, when their models are coupled with ours, required the evolution of both online (motor skill acquisition) and off-line (simulative thought rehearsal) sensorimotor prediction mechanisms within a Piagetian assimilation and accommodation framework (Wasserman & Waserman, 2016). Piaget spoke about biological maturation and interaction with the environment. He conceptualized learning and maturation through the processes of assimilation and accommodation. Herein a child processes the incoming stimuli and creates a schema. For example, four-legged creatures are "doggies." S/he then will come across animals which fit this schema, and label them accordingly, until s/he doesn't. When s/he comes across a four-legged animal and labels it "doggie," but it is what we would all agree to be a cat, the child must alter their processing and create a new schema. This latter process of accommodation allows for the incorporation, or accommodating of new material. The child of course is reinforced for correct labels, and the rewarded (declarative) behaviors and cognitive schemas become more rehearsed, often to a level of automaticity.

We are now better able to understand how this processing occurs on a neurophysiological level. Specifically, most daily behaviors are conjectured to operate automatically with rapid "online" adjustments. The adjustments are made through a process of sensorimotor anticipation, which we will explain as a combination or error analysis and reward probability assessment, the beginnings of which we have described above. The collective information remain accessible "off-line" (below conscious awareness) until the environmental stimulus that triggers their use is presented. These assessments and their paired triggers are stored in memory and are used and manipulated off-line, for the purpose of developing intentions (motivation), plans, and goals. We all see this in the increasingly sophisticated and intentional behavior of newborn to ambulatory infant behavior, reflexive to goal oriented movement, representing the development of object identification and object location, coupling with reward value.

Gweon and Schulz looked at older children within this stage. They found that 16-month-old infants can use a minimum of data about the distribution of outcomes among agents (persons) and objects to solve a fundamental inference problem. They had to cognate whether event outcomes were due to themselves or the world (agents). When infants experienced failed outcomes, their causal attributions affected whether they sought help or explored (Gweon & Schulz, 2011). This becomes important in highlighting how still within the sensorimotor stage, the infant develops from an organism relying on inborn drives and reflexes to a more purposefully ambulating and self-aware child, who is utilizing error analysis and reward probability to direct behavior and create the beginnings of a history, or physiological memory, of rewarding objects and events through the operation of cortical and subcortical network circuits.

3.2 What Is a Drive and What Is Its Relationship to Motivation?

We have written the following sentences a good many times in our work; What at first thought appears to be an easy construct to explain, turns out to be a bit less clear upon closer examination. The field of psychology is populated by terms we use with great frequency, all which we claim to understand when we are using them, and so serve as a shorthand sufficient for use in everyday language, but lack clarity and specificity when you look for a solid, agreed upon definition, for example in theory development or diagnoses. Drive is no exception. At the end, it appears that the terms drive and motivation are used interchangeably. Yet, there are some of ways to differentiate them.

There is some sense that drive refers to a set of inborn physiologically based characteristics (Deci & Ryan, 2008), while motivation refers to these same inborn characteristics modified, amplified, and differentiated as a result of a developmental course affected by cognitions and emotions derived from environmental experience. The following is an example of such a distinction; human beings have an inherent tendency to seek out novelty and challenges, to extend and exercise their capacities, to explore, and to learn. This third drive is more fragile than the other two; it needs the right environment to survive (Deci & Moller, 2005). Or this: "In our very early days, I mean very early days, say, fifty thousand years ago, the underlying assumption about human behavior was simple and true. We were trying to survive. From roaming the savannah, to gathering food, to scrambling for the bushes when a saber-toothed tiger approached, that drive guided most of our behavior. Call this early operating system Motivation 1.0. Humans are more than the sum of our biological urges. That first drive still mattered, no doubt about that, but it didn't fully account for who we are. We also had a second drive, to seek reward and avoid punishment more broadly. And it was from this insight that a new operating system, call it Motivation 2.0, arose" (Pink, 2015). Pink was referring to tangible rewards, and spoke extensively on the idea that tangible rewards could actually inhibit internal/intrinsic drive or motivation. He was therefore not a fan, and argued against external controls as they might actually serve to diminish the development of intrinsic motivation. As we will see, the neural network use of the term reward is different and far more nuanced than the strictly behaviorally oriented term: It incorporates every experience that the individual has experienced positively and has cognitive and affective components.

For our purposes, Maslow (1943) makes three notable observations about the relationship of drive to motivation. The first is that classifications of motivations must be based upon goals rather than upon instigating drives or motivated behavior. In other words, you cannot separate the motivation from its relationship to the goal. The second is that "the hunger drive (or any other physiological drive) was rejected as a centering point or model for a definitive theory of motivation. Any drive that is somatically based and localizable was shown to be atypical rather than typical in human motivation" (p. 370). We take this point to mean that motivation is far more than a purely physiological, inborn drive. The third observation is "that the situation or the field in which the organism reacts must be taken into account, but the field alone can rarely serve as an exclusive explanation for behavior. Furthermore, the field itself must be interpreted in terms of the organism" (p. 370). We understand this to mean that it is the field that can impact the development of motivation in conjunction with an inborn pattern of behaviors through the accumulation of experience. We will come back to these points frequently in our discussions as they highlight the difficulty in defining the terms as discrete entities, but are rather reflecting the involvement of the inherent drives, the attended to or selected goals and stimuli, and the unique reward history of the organism.

3.3 Stimulus Selection

How do people select from a complex array of available stimuli and related options that which they will decide to pursue. We discuss this issue extensively in the chapter on the operation of the reward network. Suffice it to say here, that people select based upon an assessment of which option has the highest reward value.

Let us begin at the beginning. The human infant has the ability to recognize facial configuration within minutes of birth. It has the ability to discriminate its primary caretaker within 6 weeks (Tzourio-Mazoyer, 2002). We note the differential motor and facial movements indicating recognition, which reinforces the caretaker, and in return reinforces the infant by insuring its survival, and through rudimentary social engagements, which are rewarding. This early interaction may well be a cornerstone of the rewarding value and motivational stepping stones of social mores.

Remember that reward value becomes very particular to each person. This reward value of the selected option is based upon a number of factors including the individual's developmental history and resultant stored probabilistic reward valuations relative to the specific goal. These reward calculations are always being assessed and modified based on new learning and experience. The selection of one action as opposed to others is also a property of the company a particular action is keeping at the proximal time. Once an individual makes this selection, the behavior they display in relation to the selected option is often considered to be representative of the construct of motivation. For example, let's assume little Bobby comes home from school one day and his mother announces that all electronics are not available during the week. Bobby has not been completing his homework, and Mom believes instituting this rule will encourage Bobby to study. Bobby can either read a book or do his homework as his mother hopes will occur. Compare this to the day before when Bobby had the opportunity to do his homework, read a book or turn on his electronics. Clearly, the electronics held the most reward value to Bobby. Mom's assumption that removing the activity of highest reward value will increase Bobby's motivation to engage in homework completion is fairly typical, albeit flawed.

For the purposes of this section, we can acknowledge that the reward possibilities of all the available options have been highly developed, automated, and stored in memory. This is because Bobby has experienced all of these options before and has made an assessment of their reward value. He can fairly reliably predict which will have the most value to him. But new information is always available, and the calculations are continuously being updated. For example, Bobbie's mother bought him a gaming magazine yesterday and it has all the updated "cheat codes" for Bobby's favorite game. The reward calculation for reading has thereby been modified (increased in value), at least in the short term.

Bobby's selection is further complicated by the issue of breadth versus depth of interest based upon prior learning (Ainley, 1987). This idea posits that Bobby might have an intense interest in one learned class of objects or experiences, such as electronics. This depth of interest is intensified over the course of development and becomes a very powerful factor in the final selection of activity. Depth is one of several attributes that plays a significant role in the determination of probabilistic reward value, in that as one gets better at some skill, hobby, interest, etc. the more one engages in that line of activity. This may be reflected in daily activities such as choosing between crossword puzzles versus Sudoku puzzles versus video coding. This may be especially true in certain clinical populations of individuals such as individuals assessed with autism spectrum disorder or individuals with obsessive compulsive disorder. Were Bobby to fall into either of these latter two categories, increasing the reward value of "doing well in class" might well fall short of the motivator necessary to increase engagement in less desirable areas. Interestingly, making the access to his electronics contingent upon homework completion might increase Bobby's desirable behavior, with Mom incorrectly concluding that she increased his motivation to do better academically. That is, motivation might have been increased, but if we are measuring it based upon grades, we would likely be measuring a latent class variable rather than "motivation" to do well on an academic task.

Returning to developmental perspectives, the developmental implications of stimulus selection are clear. From the moment of birth new information is always being encountered, and the results of that encounter are processed, stored, and subsequently available for appraisal and consideration for value calculations with future encounters with the same or highly similar objects or situations. In all circumstances the reward calculations are continuously being updated. It should be pointed out that, in some instances, the stimuli or instances are encountered so frequently that the reward calculation and subsequent selection become automated. There is really no immediate appraisal as the selection has been made so many times in the past. Think about your favorite brand of coffee. Each time you are out of coffee and you go shopping, you rather automatically reach for that brand. While you are looking for it, you are directing your attention to screen for this one brand, to the exclusion of other brands. Now, there may be time when you encounter a new brand to try, perhaps a sample provided while shopping, and you open yourself up to trying and assessing the properties of the new brand. At that moment there is a chance that your previously automated response might be changed, in the way of assimilation and accommodation processing of old schemas and new information. Think about how your trip to the supermarket would be changed if you decided to buy the new brand, in terms of active engagement in searching for a less familiar, or novel stimulus. Your search and screening process would change, and in all likelihood you would be initially less efficient and expending greater "online" energy. But if the new taste was of sufficient reward, this behavior would go on for a while, until the new choice was selected enough times to become automated.

The current authors have discussed the concept of automaticity in terms of how automated thoughts affect feeling states, and how particular automated behavioral responses may feed behavioral patterns affecting mental health (Wasserman, 2017). Here we incorporate the biological and nurtured meeting of traits: When discussing selection, we can see the beginning of how a neural network model may account for the development of traits. If an individual has an innate tendency to react to a constellation of associated stimuli in a particular way, or has learned to demonstrate a particular response in the presence of a whole complex, this response or tendency can be considered a trait. For example, infants who demonstrate a lengthy regulatory response in relation to an indication of a Moro reflex have a greater probability of developing anxiety disorders in adolescence (Goddard, 2002). This initial poor regulation and associated anxiety in relation to an initial stimulus is a tendency that the child carries forward through life and, through the process of automaticity, becomes associated with many stimuli in a schema related to anxiety. Let us return to our little Bobby for the moment. We have presented Bobby's example from a learning perspective. In order to elucidate the current point however, let us focus on the affectual rather than the reward aspects for a moment. That is, what if removing the highly rewarding stimulus, in this case access to an electronic device, resulted in emotional dysregulation rather than an easy transition across behaviors. Poor emotional accommodation would likely result in prolonged anxiety and what we would ultimately describe as a trait. This arousal trait may well in turn affect reward values and stimulus selection.

As we can see, there are now many components which contribute to development of the operational probabilistic reward calculation. The determination of selection is also based on how novel the stimulus or situation is, to what extent obtaining the target goal arouses or relieves uncertainty, to what extent acquisition of the goal arouses or relieves conflict related to the selection process, how complex the goal is, how much effort it takes to achieve the goal, and the likelihood that the pursuit of the goal will bring success. These components can be briefly defined as follows: the similarities and differences, compatibilities and incompatibilities between elements between a present stimulus and stimuli that have been experienced previously (novelty and change), between one element of a stimuli and other elements that accompany it (complexity), between simultaneously aroused responses between competing choice options (conflict), between stimuli and expectations (surprisingness), or between simultaneously aroused expectations of success (uncertainty). All of these can be considered variables in a probabilistic determination of success and the related determination of the probability of behavior to obtain a goal once it is selected. In other words, all of these, and more task specific attributes, go into the determination of how motivated or unmotivated an individual will be. As we have indicated, all of these contribute to the ever expanding schema of related reward calculations that an individual develops and retains in memory. And of course, this then drives motivation.

3.4 The Orienting Reflex

There are inborn behaviors whose principal function is to help the newborn infant interface with the environment. When an infant is presented with a novel stimulus in the environment, it orients itself to the new stimulus by becoming aroused and, at first, executing movement such as in the aforementioned rooting reflex, followed by looking in the direction of the novel thing in the environment. Later, as its motor behaviors become more complex and organized, the infant will reach for the new object to explore, and still later crawl toward the new object. Pavlov, among others, who first recognized that response, called it the orienting reflex (Pavlov, 1927). The orienting reflex is a response to a stimulus that is novel and newly encountered, in a given situation. The reflex consists of targeting, arousal and perceptual components and has three stages. These stages are represented as the movement toward the stimulus, the maintenance of fixation of the stimulus and the return movement. When the orienting reflex is evoked, perceptual learning occurs in its second stage. Pavlov considered this "reflex" as the basis of all future learning and the development of complex cognitive constructs. In this, his work presages current theories by almost 100 years.

3.5 Arousal and the Orienting Reflex

The orienting reflex includes an arousal component. This arousal component plays a significant role in the orienting reflex. The arousal level has to be sufficient enough to prepare the infant for rapid activity, should the unexpected stimulus be deemed biologically important (Zernicki, 1987). Research into the neural network function of arousal indicates that arousal states are mediated though the peripheral nervous system and neuromodulatory systems in the brainstem. Specifically, the noradrenergic nucleus locus coeruleus is activated in conjunction with the autonomic system in response to perceived biological imperatives (fight-or-flight responses). These responses can be spontaneous, occurring in relation to unexpected salient or threatening stimuli, or they can be learned responses to automated, behaviorally relevant stimuli. Noradrenaline, released in forebrain structures, facilitates sensory processing, enhances cognitive flexibility and executive function in the frontal cortex which promotes offline memory consolidation in limbic structures such as the amygdala and hippocampus. Central activation of neuromodulatory neurons and peripheral arousal together, prepare the organism for a reorientation or reset of cortical networks and the adaptive behavioral response we term arousal (Sara & Bouret, 2012).

3.6 The Arousal System in Infancy

The general arousal and integrated attention system is functional in early infancy. This system shows considerable development across infancy and early childhood with increased coordination of response developing over time. These developmental changes have a direct influence on performance, particularly on working memory tasks, in a positively correlated direction. Most importantly for our discussion, is the fact that the general arousal/attention system is nonspecific in that it functions to modulate arousal regardless of the specific task or function in which the organism is engaged. The effects of the system on arousal and attention are also general, and do not vary in a qualitative manner depending on cognitive task. Sustained attention would therefore be expected to influence recognition memory and working memory in a similar manner (Reynolds & Romano, 2016). The manner in which this system comes online, and the ease or difficulty an individual might experience in bringing it online, represents an inborn predisposition that will subsequently be modified through the life course by experience and ongoing probabilistic reward experiences as described above.

Ease of arousal clearly plays a role in the development of motivated behavior. There is a history of research that associates temperament and arousal (Trofimova & Robbins, 2016). Temperament in this regard is defined as neurochemically based individual differences in behavioral regulation. This research specifically suggests that humans possess neurochemical diversity and complexity to manage unpredictable, novel, and complex situations which entail several different psychological processes that are recruited according to prevailing contexts or states.

Currently "general arousal" theory suggests differences between two major classes of arousal: general versus localized. These two systems are sub served by different neural networks, which coexist and interact. Activities of localized arousal elements are described as being limited to basic needs behavior (food, sex, and danger-related), whereas general arousal elements influence multiple classes of behavior, and mediate both specific and nonspecific effects of arousal. Jing, Gillette, and Weiss (2009) have proposed that basic needs systems are maintained relatively independently from each other and have specific arousal systems. It is likely that these basic needs systems coexist with a very different architecture of arousal mechanism regulating the complexities of most human behavior.

Research into temperament suggests specific inborn temperamental differences in rates of arousal in infants and, subsequently, throughout the life course (Trofimova & Robbins, 2016). Specifically, this research shows the roles of noradrenaline, dopamine, and serotonin systems in mediating three complementary forms of arousal that are similar to three functional blocks described in classical models of behavior within clinical neuropsychology, psychophysiology, and temperament research. In spite of functional diversity of monoamine receptors, their functionality can be classified using three universal aspects of actions related to expansion, to selection-integration, and to maintenance of chosen behavioral alternatives. Monoamine systems also differentially regulate analytic versus routine aspects of activities at cortical and striatal neural levels. Essentially, there is an inborn, temperamental predisposition to the operation of the arousal system, and by implication, the development of motivation.

Many prominent models of emotion consider emotional arousal to reflect motivational intensity. It would be attractive to consider that the fully articulated emotional behavior of a human adult springs entirely from their arousal capabilities. This, however does not appear to be the case. According to Bradley and Lang's theory of emotion (Bradley & Lang, 2007), "judgments of arousal index (again, roughly) the degree of activation in each motivation system" (p. 585). As demonstrated by this quote, Bradley and Lang regard arousal as only a rough proxy for motivation and probably agree that arousal and motivation are not identical. There is more to the story.

How modifiable the inborn predisposition is to the operation of the reward recognition is a matter of extreme importance in the development of motivation. Life course modeling posits that human development is a lifelong processes in which individuals construct their own lives through the choices and actions they take within the opportunities and constraints of history and social circumstance (Elder, 1998). Life course modeling suggests that all of these inborn systems are modifiable systems based on the unique set of environmental interactions that occur over the life of each individual person.

3.7 Attention

We have written extensively about the role of probability reward determinations in relation to attention in general and attention deficit hyperactivity disorder (ADHD) in particular (Wasserman & Wasserman, 2015). We posited that, for individuals demonstrating symptoms associated with ADHD, their problems represented the engagement, or lack thereof, of the motivational and related reward circuit as opposed to problems, or disorders of attention traditionally defined as problems with orienting, focusing, and sustaining. We demonstrated that there is an integrated system of working memory allocation that responds by recruiting relevant aspects of both cortex and subcortex to the demands of the task being encountered. In this model, attention is viewed as a gating function determined by novelty, fight-or-flight response, and reward history/valence affecting motivation. Attention is designed to allocate working memory that is directed toward task-specific stimuli selected for interaction. The relationship to the construct of motivation is clear. Attention is the orienting and focusing operation. Motivation is what drives this function. Motivation is what causes the individual to select the stimuli of the allocation of the all-important working memory system.

There is clearly a progression of attentional skills beginning in infancy and moving onward toward adulthood. Research has demonstrated that infants with greater focused attention during memory encoding show significantly better memory performance in general and progressively better focused attention as they develop. As the authors put it, attention turns looking into seeing (Cheng, Kaldy, & Blaser, 2019). They also found that focused attention was a reliable measure of subsequent cognitive effort.

Wright and Vlietstra (1975) wrote about the developmental shift from perceptual to purposeful search behavior as a function of selective attention. They addressed the shift from perceptual exploration to logical search behavior, features which develop into the complex attention and orienting behaviors that characterize human functioning. Wright and Vlietstra posit a major developmental shift in response to the characteristics of the stimulus variables that control attending behavior. This shift describes an important contributor to the development of systematic information processing in children and makes a distinction between the constructs of exploration and search as distinctive modes of information-getting behavior. Data supports the idea that two patterns are discriminable in their own right in terms of measurable response properties. These two subtypes of attention are further discriminable in terms of the stimulus and task features that control them. They are observed to have a different course of development and period of acquisition, with exploration considered the simpler process that develops earlier than search. Exploration then, provides the germinal perceptual experiences out of which logical, systematic search can evolve when the appropriate cognitive structures for its organization become available. There is evidence that working in tandem with the developmental evolution of exploratory schemas is a shift from the control of attention by salient features of stimuli to control by logical features of the task related to that stimuli, and a shift from passively tracked, to actively sequenced attending.

3.8 Arousal and Its Relationship to Attention and Motivation

From the above, it would be possible to assume that the capacity of the individual for innate arousal would progress in a somewhat linear developmental fashion to the complex goal seeking behavior we call motivation. However, available data suggest a more complex interaction with other predisposing factors, particularly attention. This research suggests that affective states, high in motivational intensity, cause a relatively narrow attentional scope, whereas affective states low in motivational intensity, cause a relatively broad attentional scope (Gable & Jones, 2013). More specifically, states of high arousal cause a perceptual narrowing of the attentional field, while states of low arousal cause a widening of the attentional field. This, of course appears quite logical. Once aroused, an individual would narrow his focus on the object in the stimulus field that produces the most arousal. This object in the field might possess properties that are inherently interesting, such as high curiosity value, or possess properties that have developed high probabilistic reward value, or both.

Consider for example, an early wanderer in prehistory who is walking across a hill top and is attracted to a rock with an odd yellow vein in it. Driven by a combination of novelty and curiosity she picks up the rock and investigates it. She brings the rock home and throws it into a fire, and the yellow ore melts out and forms a nugget that is malleable and can make attractive objects. She wants more of these trinkets, so she goes back to the hillside to look for more of these stones. At this juncture, her arousal has focused her attention on a narrow band of stimuli; the rocks with the gold streaks. She collects several of these rocks, extracts the ore, and makes a few trinkets. No one else has them. People want them. They acquire value, and their acquisition attains probabilistic reward value thereby increasing the likelihood of continued, focused attention to this pursuit.

Also consider the more contemporary example of the co-founder of Microsoft, Bill Gates. In the popular book, *Outliers* (Gladwell, 2008), Malcolm Gladwell outlines the intense interest and corresponding effort Gates put into pursuing his "obsession." This biographical material includes an account of a single 7 month period in which time Gates and his friends put in 1575 h of computer time, which comes to 8 h a day, 7 days a week. At the age of 15 he would take the bus to the University of Washington to work on their computer between the hours of 3 and 6 am. We are all likely aware of the trajectory of his interests culminating in the software giant Microsoft.

On the other hand, lack of arousal would, as indicated, lead to an expanding of the stimulus field so that the individual can find more things in which to be interested. It would be more precise to say that complex human motivation arises from a multivariate set of inborn predispositions including ease of arousal, curiosity, attentional regulation, and novelty at the least, in conjunction with external variables such as access. Each individual would possess a unique combination of these variables which would all vary in frequency, intensity, and duration of expression across and in response to internal and external stimuli.

3.9 Boredom

While this is a book on motivation, not boredom, it is important to understand that, from a neural network perspective, boredom and motivation are understood utilizing the same probabilistic modeling. The two constructs represent points along a common distribution. In this regard, one way to think about boredom is that it represents a state of being that is the opposite of being motivated. Failing to find anything of interest, based upon internal variables, an individual remains in a state of low arousal and is now officially bored. Another way that boredom can be characterized is as a low state of arousal secondary to a stimulus field absent of externally attractive targets.

A model of boredom based on neural network understanding would say that boredom represents a low state of arousal and related goal seeking behavior that is on a continuum, with the upper end representing high motivation. This, however, is not the only way that a network work model may describe boredom. There are models that conjecture an interplay between arousal and directed attention as causative to the creation of boredom. These models suggest that when people have high arousal, they have energy they would like to devote to something, but they cannot find anything engaging. This results in boredom (Eastwood, Frischen, Fenske, & Smilek, 2012). Specifically, they suggest that boredom is definable in relation to attention. That is, boredom is the aversive state that occurs when individuals "(a) are not able to successfully engage attention with internal (e.g., thoughts or feelings) or external (e.g., environmental stimuli) information required for participating in satisfying activity, (b) are focused on the fact that we are not able to engage attention and participate in satisfying activity, and (c) attribute the cause of our aversive state to the environment" (p. 482). In other words, these models would imply that people who were bored were, in fact, reportedly motivated to do something, but not able to identify what it was that they wanted to do.

Thus, boredom would differ from motivation in terms of the arousal and attentional focus of having a task or goal which could narrow focus and direct behavior. Motivated people would have one, bored people wouldn't. This would imply that the physiological and attentional readiness that are important preconditions for motivation cannot occur in the absence of a goal and would therefore not result in motivated behavior. Or, to state it in another way, motivation only happens in response to a specific goal or circumstance. These goals and circumstances would be identified and catalogued through interaction and feedback with the environment over time.

For completeness sake, we will note that there are nonneural network models that have been proffered to explain boredom. These models separate to some extent, the two constructs of boredom and motivation. Arousal theories define boredom as the state of nonoptimal arousal that occurs when there is a disconnect between an individual's needed arousal and the availability of environmental stimulation. More specifically, the environment may present too much or too little challenge, and thus does not afford the possibility of engaging in a satisfying activity (Berlyne, 1960). Cognitive theories focus on the individuals' perception of their environment as monotonous or uninteresting (Fisher, 1993; Hill & Perkins, 1985). Cognitive theories of boredom stress that bored individuals suffer from poor concentration, and are forced to control their attention with effort (Todman, 2003). We understand this to mean that the person in question is perceiving their environment as lacking, perhaps reflective of an inability to apply their energy in a particular direction. In sum, the definition of boredom from a cognitive perspective emphasizes both attributions; the environment lacking opportunities for satisfying activity, as well as the individual's impaired ability to concentrate.

There are models of boredom that suggest boredom is the state of natural motivation being impeded. For example, there is research to suggest that boredom signals a motivational state characterized by high anxious uncertainty coupled with low approach motivation that is conducive to self-control failure (Britton, 2018). It is also clear that boredom has some positive aspects associated with it in addition to the negative ones that are typically identified. For example, boredom may prompt the search for more satisfying activity (Bench & Lench, 2013).

3.10 Adaptive and Defensive Reaction

Adaptive and defensive reactions center on the idea that evolution has provided all living organisms, including humans, with an inborn set of responses in order to avoid a wide range of ecological dangers (Bolles & Fanselow, 1980). The best known of these is the fight-or-fight response. Models have described two general classes of adaptive and defensive responses: those that occur when the danger is distant and those that occur when the danger is close. Models that have been developed to describe the neural network properties of these various reactions have posited that when a distant threat is confronted, specialized higher cortico-limbic regions including the ventral medial prefrontal cortex mPFC (vmPFC) and hippocampus gather contingency and contextual information and, via the amygdala, instigate survival actions by controlling midbrain systems [e.g., ventrolateral periaqueductal gray (PAG)] evoked freezing. The network properties of the response to close threats are somewhat different. Imminent threat corresponds with the inhibition of forebrain circuits, with midbrain regions such as the dorsolateral PAG becoming dominant, which, in turn, engineer active defense reactions (e.g., fight or flight). It is from these inherent responses, common to all animals including humans, that the highly complex and cognitively infused defensive responses that characterize human beings are developed.

3.11 Exploratory Behavior: Locomotor Exploration

Exploratory locomotion represents an innate reflex that, in part, serves as one of the essential building blocks for the development of motivation (Berlyne, 1960). It is a more complex behavior than a simple rooting reflex or moro reflex. Exploratory locomotion now incorporates attention variables and object location which permits the infant to survey its new environment. Based initially upon novelty, the infant is expressing curiosity-based behaviors.

At first glance, exploratory locomotion does not seem to fit neatly into a probabilistic model. However, let us remember the difference between exploratory behavior and search behavior. In fact, exploratory behavior is seen across the mammalian spectrum and presents very early on. The exploratory pattern of behavior is limited initially, restricted by the limited coordination of the human infant. As the cerebral-muscular-skeletal system becomes better integrated, locomotion becomes extended and expressed with greater intent. Exploratory locomotion then initially follows the pattern of inborn reflexes that are activated by stimuli with specific physicochemical properties and gives rise to uniform response sequences. Through this exploratory locomotion, both curiosity and reward variables continue to become more sophisticated and integrated.

First and foremost, although the drive to explore may be innate, the objects chosen for exploration must have properties that attract the infant to them. These properties are, in fact, the same ones we have alluded to previously. For the most part, early on the two main properties are probably either novelty or familiarity. There is research to suggest that early on infants prefer familiar stimuli. At 6 weeks of age infants fixate on familiar objects significantly more than on novel objects. This difference disappears at 8 weeks and the direction of the difference is, in fact reversed, resulting in a preference for novel stimuli (Weizmann, Cohen, & Pratt, 1971). It is likely that some preference for the familiar remains, depending upon the circumstances. However, novelty is a major source of drive for the newly ambulating infant.

To state that the exploration of novel stimuli is an inborn human predisposition is to state that the exploration of the novel is one of the foundations of what comes to be known as motivation. It is fairly straightforward to understand how this might be so. The infant, in its early exploration of novel stimuli and environments, encounters success or frustration. Success would reinforce the temperamental predisposition, and failure would inhibit its expression. Infants who encountered success and support would produce the behavior at a higher rate. Infants that received discouragement or received failure would have the response rate inhibited. With the imposition of cognitive descriptors and controls, successful individuals would become "motivated." Inhibited individuals would not. Task specificity would play a role, unless an individual youngster was uniformly inhibited, and specific areas of competencies would develop. Let us suppose that there were brothers whose parents noticed something in their early behavior that indicated that one was "academically inclined" and one was "good with his hands" and could build things. They were provided early and continuous experiences early on. One brother believed that academic tasks were easy, and the other came to find building things enjoyable. Both were competent in their respective selected endeavors. They each became motivated toward activities representative of the early programming. They each found the other interests unmotivating. Both brothers started in the same place temperamentally, and were shaped by life course events into the motivated individuals they became as adults.

3.12 Exploratory Behavior: Investigatory Responses

To this point, the types of responses we have been discussing, orienting responses and locomotor exploration, effect changes in the person in response to an environmental stimulus. The stimulus is unaltered. In the case of investigatory behavior, this relationship does not hold. Investigative responses imply that the individual manipulates or modifies some as aspect of the environment and learns from the result. There is one feature of investigatory behavior that has significant impact. This is the fact that an organism that is effecting changes in external objects as a way of modifying the stimuli reaching its own receptors is simultaneously modifying the stimulus field for any other organism that is in the vicinity. Human investigatory behavior includes much of the creative activity on which science, art, and entertainment depend (Berlyne, 1960).

There is some suggestion that investigatory behavior is initially innate (Mongomery, 2019). This research posits that curiosity, experimentation, and ultimately creativity are inborn uniquely to each human being. These inborn predispositions are shaped by life course factors and develop into the complex human behaviors that govern complex human exploration.

There is much to recommend in this model. As far as motivation goes, it would argue that inborn curiosity and the desire to explore were developed by these inborn predispositions interacting with and receiving feedback from the environment. They would contribute to the development of complex goal seeking behavior.

At first glance, this model of development would appear to argue for consideration of motivation derived from exploratory behavior being a trait. Initially an individual is either more or less disposed to explore, or more or less innately curious. While this could be true, it is equally likely that these inborn predispositions are shaped in response to more limited classes of stimuli. That given the usual successes and failure that occur with regularity over the life course and an individual's curiosity, exploration and resulting exploration would be focused on classes of skills as opposed to every skill.

3.13 Critical Thinking and Motivation

What happens when we have a problem, and no solution is readily apparent? Perhaps the problem blocks the pathway toward a goal or perhaps there are multiple pathways available and we haven't had the experience necessary to decide which pathway to follow. In the most general sense, "a problem arises when we have a goal, a state of affairs that we want to achieve, and it is not immediately apparent how the goal can be attained?" Psychologists have studied this phenomenon under the terms problem solving or critical thinking. Neural network modeling would argue that motivation is a key component of this activity. In order to be able to think critically, it is required that a person feel motivated to choose a particular alternative. In order for this to occur there must be a clear and identifiable path to follow and that this path have both a high probability of being accomplished and a high probability that the goal would be obtained. From a developmental perspective, how would we acquire the ability to maintain motivation in the many circumstances where these conditions for success were not established?

Critical thinking includes a number of component skills including analyzing arguments, making inferences using inductive or deductive reasoning, judging or evaluating, and making decisions or solving problems. Background knowledge is a necessary but not a sufficient condition for enabling critical thought within a given subject. Critical thinking involves both cognitive skills and what have been termed in the critical thinking literature, dispositions. These dispositions can be thought of as attitudes or habits of mind, include open and fair-mindedness, inquisitiveness, flexibility, a propensity to seek reason, a desire to be well informed, and a respect for and willingness to entertain diverse viewpoints. There are both general- and domain-specific aspects of critical thinking (Lai, 2011).

3.14 Dispositions/Motivation

Research demonstrates that in addition to skills or abilities, critical thinking also involves dispositions (Facione, 2000). Unsurprisingly, the ability to think critically is distinct from the disposition to do so. Critical thinking abilities and dispositions are, in fact, separate entities. Dispositions have variously been described as attitudes or habits of mind, which are consistent internal motivations to act toward or respond to persons, events, or circumstances in habitual, yet potentially modifiable ways. In other words, dispositions represent motivation. So how is motivation developed and associated with critical thinking?

While working on the problem, individuals have to assess the quality of their performance: Are they getting closer to the goal or not? (Davidson & Sternberg, 2003). In addition, research has identified experiential and mood-related elements to the process. Not only is it important to identify that one is making progress toward the goal. In the absence of progress it is possible to maintain motivation by enjoying the experience of problem solving itself. Individuals that enjoy working on challenging problems will work on the problems because of the challenge itself. It is not difficult to see how this might occur. Novelty and exploratory drive may impel initial exploratory behavior which, in and of itself, rewarding. It would be clear that individuals who experience this state and then went on to solve problems would be rewarded for their efforts and be more likely to continue this behavior in the future. On the other hand, even if the exploratory and novelty were sufficient to initiate motivation, if no resolution were ever reached it is likely that problem solving would become associated with frustration. In this instance, problem solving may lose it motivational value in a probabilistic reward value calculation.

3.15 Skills

Motivation for critical thinking can be developed and maintained through the teaching of basic problem solving skills and the achievement of mastery (Mayer, 1998). In this regard, metacognitive skill training in general problems solving skills seems to be an important component in problem solving. This involves knowledge of when to use, how to coordinate, and how to monitor various skills in problem solving.

3.16 Interest

Interest can be either based on previous, successful and enjoyable interaction with the general subject matter that is related to the specific problem or novelty. We have seen how both of these fit comfortably within a neural network consideration. Interest theory predicts that individuals will think harder and process more diligently when they are interested rather than uninterested. Unsurprisingly, there is considerable research to support this conjecture (Schiefele, Krapp, & Winteler, 1992).

3.17 The Reduction of Conflict

We have mentioned internal, value-based conflict as one source of input to develop motivation. Conflict occurs in many ways. There can be competition for choice selection, confusion about the best possible choice, a determination of which choice has the least painful negative outcomes, or a determination of which choice represents the best moral choice, to name a few. Increased conflict amongst goals has deleterious effects on motivation and other emotional states. For example, implicit goal conflict itself has been found to cause negative affect (Chartrand & Bargh, 2002) and decreased desirability for the target goal (Aarts, Custers, & Holland, 2007). These conflicts cause individuals to become anxious and uncertain. The resolution/reduction of conflict increases motivation by reducing uncertainty and anxiety. The closer various options are to each other in terms of valuation, the greater the possibility of conflict among a few desirable options. This would lead to anxiety, uncertainty, and less motivation. The clearer the winning choice is, the less conflict among choices exists, and the greater the motivation is for the selected choice. Reducing conflict through the experience of competing choices increases the motivation for the winning choices over time.

There can be incompatibilities between various symbolic responses, such as ideas, that do not represent tangible items. Berlyne (1960) termed these as cognitive conflicts. These are resolved in a similar fashion as conflicts representing tangible choices. The value of the ideas, and the resulting actions related to them, are assessed and acted upon. The power of the various cognitions, such as ideas and values to drive behavior, develop and change through experience.

3.18 Arousal Potential, Perceptual Curiosity and Learning

Arousal potential is the innate capability of a stimulus to induce arousal in any person, independent of that person's experience with the stimulus. It is the difference between a Ferris wheel at the state fair and a blade of grass that the Ferris wheel is sitting on. Given curiosity and novelty alone, one has, at least for most people, a significantly higher innate capacity to produce arousal. Research has clearly demonstrated a predictable relationship between arousal potential and actual arousal (Steenkamp, Baumgartner, & der Wulpb, 1996). As we have indicated this innate potential is modified, amplified or reduced by the effects of environmental interaction and learning. This shaping process is idiosyncratic to the individual as are the resulting motivational properties of the original stimuli.

The relation between arousal and arousal potential can be impacted by a number of factors. When arousal potential is very low, arousal may actually rise. As we have shown, an environment with exceptionally low simulative properties may cause the upsurge of arousal that characterizes boredom. Just think of what might happen if you were placed in an all-white room for example. In other situations, as when the intensity of a stimulus falls almost to the threshold as compared to several other available stimuli, there will likely be an increase of arousal due to conflict. The point of this being that arousal potential of an object or experience may in initially solely the property of the object or experience but is modified through experience to be idiosyncratically arousing/ motivating to each individual.

3.19 Summary

A neural network model of motivation would, in line with many other theories of motivation, insist that all behavior is motivated. It is commonly taken to mean that every piece of behavior can be traced to a particular drive or combination of drives (Berlyne, 1960). Heckhausen and Heckhausen (2008) concluded their extensive review of motivation by identifying many of the factors that would contribute to the term "combination of drives." They stated that an individual's motivation to pursue a certain goal is the cumulative result of situational stimuli, personal preferences, and the interaction of the two. The resultant motivational tendency is a composite of the various incentives associated with the activity, its outcome, and its internal (self-evaluative) and external consequences, each weighted according to their own personal motive. This interpretation is entirely consistent with a neural network model based on probabilistic reward conceptualizations.

To the above, from a network perspective, we would add that each of these factors develops from a base collection of inborn predisposing temperamental tendencies that include arousal, curiosity, attention, novelty, adaptive, and defensive reactions all developed along a unique path shaped by life course experiences and the probabilistic reward valuations that result from them. In addition, far from being a trait, motivation has many state-like properties. The individual's ability to demonstrate motivation is highly dependent on the task, the individual's history with the task and how closely a new task approximates tasks and the associated probabilistic reward valences that the individual has already stored in memory.

References

Aarts, H., Custers, R., & Holland, R. W. (2007). The nonconscious cessation of goal pursuit: When goals and negative affect are coactivated. *Journal of Personality and Social Psychology, 92*, 165–178. https://doi.org/10.1037/0022-3514.92.2.165.

Aboitz, F. M. (2003). The evolutionary origin of the mammalian isocortex: Toward an integrated developmental and functional approach. *The Behavioral and Brain Sciences, 26*, 535–552.

Ainley, M. (1987). The factor structure of curiosity measures: Breadth and depth of interest curiosity styles. *Australian Journal of Psychology, 39*(1), 53–59.

Bench, S. W., & Lench, H. C. (2013). On the function of boredom. *Behavioral Sciences, 3*, 459–472. https://doi.org/10.3390/bs3030459.

Berlyne, D. (1960). *Conflict, arousal, and curiosity*. New York: McGraw-Hill. https://doi.org/10.1037/11164-000.

Bolles, R., & Fanselow, M. (1980). A perceptual-defensive-recuperative model of fear and pain. *Behavioral and Brain Science, 3*, 291–301.

Bradley, M., & Lang, P. (2007). Emotion and motivation. In J. Cacioppo, L. Tassinary, & G. Berntson (Eds.), *Handbook of psychophysiology* (pp. 581–607). New York: Cambridge University Press.

Britton, E. (2018). *Boredom and motivation: From anxious uncertainty and low approach motivation to low self control.* University of Waterloo. Retrieved from https://uwspace.uwaterloo.ca/bitstream/handle/10012/13680/Britton_Emily.pdf?sequence=3&isAllowed=y.

Chartrand, T. L., & Bargh, J. A. (2002). Nonconscious motivations: Their activation, operation, and consequences. In A. Tesser & D. Stapel (Eds.), *Self and motivation: Emerging psychological perspectives* (pp. 13–41). Washington, DC: American Psychological Association. https://doi.org/10.1037/10448-001.

Cheng, C., Kaldy, Z., & Blaser, E. (2019). Focused attention predicts visual working memory performance in 13-month-old infants: A pupillometric study. *Developmental Cognitive Neuroscience, 36*, 100616. https://doi.org/10.1016/j.dcn.2019.100616.

Davidson, J., & Sternberg, R. (2003). *The psychology of problem solving*. New York: Cambridge University Press.

Deci, E., & Moller, A. (2005). TThe concept of competence: A starting place for understanding intrinsic motivation and self-determined extrinsic motivation. In A. Elliot & C. Dweck (Eds.), *Handbook of competence and motivation* (pp. 579–595). New York: Guilford.

Deci, E. L., & Ryan, R. M. (2008). Self-determination theory: A macrotheory of human motivation, development, and health. *Canadian Psychology/Psychologie Canadienne, 49*(3), 182–185.

Eastwood, J., Frischen, A., Fenske, M., & Smilek, D. (2012). The unengaged mind: Defining boredom. *Perspectives on Psychological Science, 7*(5), 482–495. https://doi.org/10.1177/1745691612456044.

Elder, G. (1998). The life course as developmental theory. *Child Development, 69*(1), 1–12.

Facione, P. (2000). The disposition toward critical thinking: Its character, measurement, and relation to critical thinking skill. *Informal Logic, 20*(1), 61–84.

Fisher, C. (1993). Boredom at work: A neglected concept. *Human Relations, 46*, 395–417.

Gable, P., & Jones, E. (2013). These results suggest that affective states high in on attentional scope and the late positive potential? *Psychophysiology, 50*, 344–350. https://doi.org/10.1111/psyp.12023.

Gladwell, M. (2008). *Outliers*. New York: Little, Brown.
Goddard, S. (2002). *Moro reflex*. Neuroclinicbarrie. Retrieved from http://wp-content/uploads/2018/06/suzanne-day_reflexes-learning-behavior.pdf.
Gweon, H., & Schulz, L. (2011). 16-Month-olds rationally infer causes of failed actions. *American Association for the Advancement of Science (AAAS), 332*, 1524. https://doi.org/10.1126/science.1204493.
Heckhausen, J., & Heckhausen, H. (2008). *Motivation and action* (2nd ed.). New York: Cambridge University Press.
Hill, A. B., & Perkins, R. E. (1985). Towards a model of boredom. *British Journal of Psychology, 76*, 235–240.
Jing, J., Gillette, R., & Weiss, K. (2009). Evolving concepts of arousal: Insights from simple model systems. *Reviews in the Neurosciences, 20*(5–6), 405–427.
Koziol, L., & Budding, D. (2009). *Subcortical structures and cognition: Implications for neuropsychological assessment*. New York: Springer.
Koziol, L., & Budding, D. (2009). *Subcortical structures and cognition Springer International Publishing*. ISBN 978-0-387-84868-6.
Koziol, L., Budding, D., & Chidekel, D. (2012). From movement to thought: Executive function, embodied cognition, and the cerebellum. *Cerebellum, 11*(2), 505–525. https://doi.org/10.1007/s12311-011-0321-y.
Lai, E. (2011, June). *Critical thinking: A literature review*. Retrieved from pearsonassessments.com: http://images.pearsonassessments.com/images/tmrs/CriticalThinkingReviewFINAL.pdf.
Maslow, A. H. (1943). A theory of human motivation. *Psychological Review, 50*(4), 370–396.
Mayer, R. (1998). Cognitive, metacognitive, and motivational aspects of problem solving. *Instructional Science, 26*, 49–63.
McLeod, S. A. (2009, April 9). *Simply psychology*. Sensorimotor stage. Retrieved from https://www.simplypsychology.org/sensorimotor.html.
Middleton, F. S. (2000). Basal ganglia output and cognition: Evidence from anatomical, behavioral and clinical studies. *Brain and Cognition, 42*, 183–200.
Mongomery, J. (2019). *Innate painting : Investigating of origins of artistic production through connections between curiosity experimentation and creativity*. US Space instituional Repository. Retrieved from https://repository.up.ac.za/handle/2263/70429.
Pavlov, I. (1927). *Varieties of exploratory behavior; the orientation reaction; functions of the orientation reaction; dynamics of the orientation reaction; adaptive and defensive reaction; the orientation reaction and arousal; the orientation reaction and orienting respons*. Oxford: Oxford University Press.
Piaget, J., & Inhelder, B. (1972). *The psychology of the child*. London: Routledge.
Pink, D. (2015). *Drive: The surprising truth about what motivates us*. The Sage School. Retrieved from https://thesageschool.org/wp-content/uploads/Drive-by-Daniel-Pink.pdf.
Reynolds, G., & Romano, A. (2016). The development of attention systems and working memory in infancy. *Frontiers in Systems. Neuroscience, 10*, Article 15. https://doi.org/10.3389/fnsys.2016.00015.
Saint-Cyr, J. (2003). Frontal striatal circuit functions: Context, sequence and consequence. *Journal of the International Neuropsychology Society, 9*, 103–127.
Sara, S., & Bouret, S. (2012). Orienting and reorienting: The locus coeruleus mediates cognition through arousal. *Neuron, 76*(1), 130–141. https://doi.org/10.1016/j.neuron.2012.09.011.
Schiefele, U., Krapp, A., & Winteler, A. (1992). Interest as a predictor of academic achievement: A meta-analysis of research. In K. Renninger, S. Hidi, & A. Krapp (Eds.), *The role of interest in learning and development* (pp. 182–313). Hillsdale, NJ: Erlbaum.
Steenkamp, J.-B., Baumgartner, J., & der Wulpb, E. (1996). The relationships among arousal potential, arousal and stimulus evaluation, and the moderating role of need for stimulation. *International Journal of Research in Marketing, 13*(4), 319–329. https://doi.org/10.1016/S0167-8116(96)00013-4.
Todman, M. (2003). Boredom and psychotic disorders: Cognitive and motivational issues. *Psychiatry, 66*, 146–167.

Trofimova, I., & Robbins, T. (2016). Temperament and arousal systems: A new synthesis of differential psychology and functional neurochemistry. *Neuroscience and Biobehavioral Reviews, 64*, 382–402. https://doi.org/10.1016/j.neubiorev.2016.03.008.

Tzourio-Mazoyer, N. D. (2002). Neural correlates of woman face processing by 2-month-old infants. *NeuroImage, 15*, 454–461.

Wasserman, T., & Waserman, L. (2016). *Depathologizing psychopathology*. New York: Springer.

Wasserman, T., & Wasserman, L. (2015). The misnomer of attention deficit hyperactivity disorder. *Applied Neuropsychology: Child, 4*(2), 116–122. https://doi.org/10.1080/21622965.2015.1005487.

Wasserman, T. W. (2017). *Neurocognitive learning therapy: Theory and practice*. Cham: Springer.

Weizmann, F., Cohen, L., & Pratt, J. (1971). Novelty, familiarity, and the development of infant attention. *Developmental Psychology, 4*(2), 149–154.

Wright, J., & Vlietstra, A. (1975). The development of selective attention: From perceptual exploration to logical search. *Advances in Child Development and Behavior, 10*, 195–239. https://doi.org/10.1016/S0065-2407(08)60011-7.

Zernicki, B. (1987). Pavlovian orienting reflex. *Acta Neurobiologiae Experimentalis, 47*, 239–247.

Chapter 4
The Role of the Reward Recognition Network in Understanding Motivation

If we are to understand a truly complex construct such as motivation in terms of its operation over neural networks, then it is imperative to elucidate how combinations of neural network functions allow a human to pursue a specific goal to the exclusion of others. In fact, it is imperative to keep in mind that the process requires the interconnectedness of multiple network systems. There are then, a number of networks that make contributions to this process, including networks responsible for error predictions and adjustments, emotional respondency, memory, and the one responsible for reward recognition. This chapter is about the reward recognition network and its role in the creation of "motivated behavior" in human beings.

There are specific aspects of learning, about which rewards we determine to be of value to us, that are directly related to the development of motivation. Since all events have the potential of being rewarding, some more so than others, how do we go through this complex process of determining the "worth" or reward value of any event or object or experience? Furthermore, how does this determination of worth figure into the operation of motivation? This happens when the determination of worth that is recorded in memory is used by the individual to anticipate worth the next time the stimulus is encountered. This concept of reward anticipation includes cue evaluation, motor preparation, and feedback anticipation (Zhang, Wang, Li, Liu, & Zhen, 2017). The process itself is also tied to effort expenditure. Yi, Mei, Zhang, and Zheng (2020) found support for the idea that the amount of effort expenditure reduces reward sensitivity during the anticipatory phase and enhances reward sensitivity during the consummatory phase. That is, for any given task or goal driven behavior, the amount of effort needed impacts our "motivation" to secure the said goal. Subsequently, attaining the goal sucessfully increases its valence. Long-term memory mechanisms related to the recognition of reward must balance the need to represent potential determinants of all available reward outcomes with the computational burden of an over-inclusive memory and limited working memory capacity (Murty and Adcock, 2014).

T. Wasserman, L. Wasserman, *Motivation, Effort, and the Neural Network Model*, Neural Network Model: Applications and Implications,
https://doi.org/10.1007/978-3-030-58724-6_4

Remembering that reward value in a positive mode would likely increase future efforts in that direction, how then might the process be facilitated. One solution would be to enhance memory for specific salient events that occur during reward anticipation. The memory enhancement would likely have emotional saliency, and this has in fact been demonstrated by research indicating that reward motivation can enhance hippocampus-dependent memory and anticipatory ventral tegmental area (VTA)-cortical–hippocampal interactions (Ranganath, 2010). Other research demonstrates the dopaminergic neuromodulation of prefrontal function and hippocampus-dependent memory (Berridge & Robinson, 1998).

In sum, once reward value is established, we engage in a constant process of evaluating rewards, reassessing reward valuation and determining whether or not to engage. One possible way to understand motivation is to understand how one signal becomes more amplified, attention regulating and behaviorally regulating than others. This speaks to the reward salience of the target. There are candidates for how this might occur. Included in these candidates are the ideas that the context of the signal in the environment modulates signal strength. Another candidate is that error analysis or error prediction, an ongoing process is constantly modulating signal strength. One way the neural network might operationalize this process is for VTA modulation to induce distributed neural changes that amplify hippocampal signals. Another way is for memory to record the impact of expectancy violations which modify saliency. That is, the process involves and includes history, working memory, and attached emotional value.

The above is just one way to understand how the reward network plays a crucial role in the expression of motivated behavior. As we will see below, there are many other ways this important network contributes. Using our understanding of this and other key networks, it will be possible to build a model that will explain how motivation operates in the human brain.

4.1 Some Background on Neural Networks

Perhaps one of the hardest paradigm shifts to accept is that complex human behavior can be explained with a neural network model. How do we shift from believing that the "whole is greater than the sum of its parts" to what seems to be a reductionist model? It is important to remember that neural networks include emotional and personal memory aspects (Wasserman & Wasserman, 2017). Neural networks are the future and past repositories of all that makes us both human and unique. Therefore, while certain classes of tasks may recruit certain cortical structures and regions across persons, as components of their particular network, each network is task-specific and in some way unique to each person. This can be perhaps better imagined by looking at neural imaging studies across subjects; some common areas are recruited, but scatter, or personal variations exist. The neural network combinations involved in any particular task or experience are however mappable, with some commonalities, and some unique variations.

To reiterate an important concept; at its core, a neural network, or circuit, is simply a population of neurons located throughout the brain that are interconnected by synapses. These neurons are interconnected by the brain in a task-dependent manner to carry out certain specific functions. Each new task that a person faces causes the creation of a network to solve it. Deciding which task to solve involves is based on a number of factors that essentially comprise what we will come to call motivation. These include factors based in history such as, how much do I like what will happen if I solve this task or engage in this activity, how likely is it that I will actually be able to do what is required and how much effort will I have to expend to do what is required.

There are, however, tasks and situations that recur frequently. These cause the creation of collections of neurons and structures that have purposes that are constantly being utilized by a functioning brain. These can be recognizable as known networks because the demands of the tasks require skills to solve them that are common or shared across persons. One of these networks is the reward recognition network, and it is utilized to learn about, store, remember, and recall environmental stimuli that were rewarding for the person. That is the essence of what it does. The relationship of this function to a construct-like motivation has to be established by connecting the function of the network to the operation of the construct. As we have seen above, we can model just such a connection, and begin to discuss how the recognition of rewards contributes to the development of motivation.

4.2 Network Structures of Reward

As discussed above, analyzing, predicting or anticipating reward involves a number of brain networks specifically recruited to meet the processing requirements of the task at hand. Central to them all, is the fronto-striatal neural circuit, which is a core component of every operation of the reward system (Haber & Knutson, 2010). This fronto-striatal circuit involves dopaminergic projections from midbrain nuclei (e.g., the ventral tegmental area) to subcortical regions that process the rewarding properties of stimuli (e.g., the ventral striatum, including the nucleus accumbens) to cortical target regions (e.g., the orbitofrontal cortex, medial prefrontal cortex, anterior cingulate cortex). This circuit, when functioning as part of an anticipatory process, is responsible, in part for a process that includes reward-responsivity, incentive-based learning, assessing probability of reward receipt, prediction error, and goal-directed behavior (Nusslock & Alloy, 2017). In fact, in both the processes of downregulation or upregulation, the cellular responses (increases or decreases in responsivity) to a stimulus such as insulin, or drug addiction, have been shown to occur in the brain regions such as the nucleus accumbens (Nestler, 2014), which is a component of the fronto-striatal network in these sort of situations.

4.3 Neural Networks and Behavioral Regulation

An important finding of Browne et al. (2020) is that network regulatory process, such as are often described as executive functions, appear to be sensitive to both external stimuli and an epigenetic influence. That is, what develop into fairly stable epigenetic mechanisms are continuously influenced by external factors, e.g., drugs or hormones, and in turn, the resulting epigenetic mechanisms control behavioral responses to the drug or hormone, on a cellular level. Questions remain as to how this functionally occurs. These questions might include whether these changes relate to the constructs of reward and, by extension, motivation, and these changes can become transgenerational thereby impacting next generation developmental aspects of motivation or reward sensitivity.

Returning to our discussion of reward processing networks, a number of brain structures along these network lines are thought to be involved in specific aspects of reward processing, specifically anticipation vs. attainment or consumption. While anticipation, attainment, and consumption all occur as part of a process of obtaining and utilizing a reward, the processing requirement for each of these "phases" are somewhat different. The core reward networks would be used for all of them, but other networks would be recruited depending on the task demands of the phase of the overall reward process. For example, anticipation of rewards activates a broad network, including the medial frontal cortex and ventral striatum. Attainment of reward also activates memory and emotion-related regions such as the hippocampus and parahippocampal gyrus, but not the ventral striatum. Reward consumption, in contrast, is associated with amygdala activation and under some conditions, the thalamus. (Kal, Case, Freed, Stern, & Gabbay, 2017). Therefore, the available research suggests dissociable neural networks for the anticipation and/vs. attainment of reward. In addition, there are some findings that the neural mechanisms underlying reward consumption are in fact more modality-specific than those for reward anticipation, and that they are mediated by subjective reward value (Rademacher et al., 2010). For example, Rademacher et al. (2010) found differential activations for social reward versus monetary reward in the attainment phase, with the amygdala and thalamus reacting respectively. Putting this into perspective, these finding of activation of a broader network during the anticipation phase makes sense as the process at this stage involves a more subjective analysis, involving a wider range of outcomes, with each containing a potential reward value.

As related phenomenon, we look at positive prediction error (PPE), defined as the attainment of an unexpected gain or reward, activated an entirely different network. PPE activated a right-dominant fronto-temporo-parietal network (Kal et al., 2017). This indicated, as we would suspect, that there is an analysis component to prediction errors designed to correct and modify future analyses.

Finally, "Converging data demonstrate two parallel neural networks within the Prefrontal Cortex (PFC); one, including the dorsolateral PFC (DLPFC), involved in working memory (WM) and planning, and the other, including the ventral PFC (VPFC) and to some extent the ventral medial areas (MPFC), associated with reward sensitivity and motivation" (Pochon et al., 2002. (p. 5669).

How then do we tie this body of information regarding the human's ability to recognize and analyze reward to the construct of motivation, which concerns itself with the power of goal-directed activity? It is to that issue we now turn our attention.

4.4 Network Anatomy of Value-Based Decision-Making in the Human Brain

Neuroimaging studies have identified the neural networks activated by value estimations and choice behavior in humans. For the purposes of discussion, value can be considered the estimation of how rewarding a particular choice is perceived.

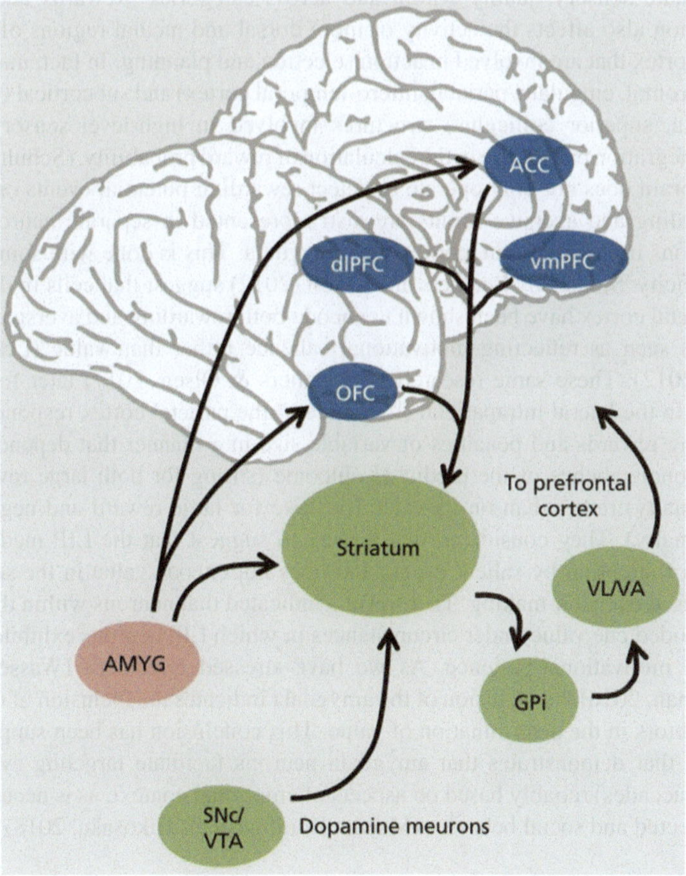

Simplified schematic representation of the reward and decision-making network. Midbrain nuclei containing dopaminergic neurons: *AMYG* amygdala, *GPi* internal globus pallidus, *SNc/VTA* substantia nigra pars compacta/ventral tegmental area, *VL/VA* ventral lateral and anterior thalamic nuclei. Subdivisions of the prefrontal cortex: *ACC* anterior cingulate cortex, *dlPFC* dorsolateral prefrontal cortex, *OFC* orbitofrontal cortex, *vmPFC* ventromedial prefrontal cortex (Sirigu & Duhamel, 2016)

Reward-related behavior emerges from the dynamic activity of entire neural networks rather than from any single brain structure (Kelley & Berridge, 2002). Specific reward signals are found in most midbrain dopamine neurons, as well as in subsets of neurons receiving dopaminergic projections in the orbitofrontal cortex (OFC), in the ventral striatum, and in the amygdala. These neurons also respond to conditioned stimuli that serve to predict future reward. Other cells connect information about reward with sensory or action information. These are also neurons that discriminate sensory quality within and across categories. Rewards and reward expectation also affects the activity of more dorsal and medial regions of the prefrontal cortex that are involved in action selection and planning. In fact, many cortical (prefrontal, cingulate, parietal, infero-temporal cortex) and subcortical (striatum, amygdala, superior colliculus) structures involved in high-level sensory and/or motor integration participate in the calculation of reward probability. (Schultz, 2015).

The brain does not only operate to detect rewarding potential events or stimuli. Unrewarding and aversive events are also represented in separate neuronal subpopulations in the midbrain, cortex, and amygdala. This is done with some degree of specificity. Studies by Leathers and Olson (2012) suggest that cells in the posterior parietal cortex have been shown to encode both rewarding and aversive stimuli, which is seen as reflecting motivational salience rather than value (Leathers & Olson, 2012). These same researchers (Leathers & Olsen, 2017) later found that neurons in the lateral intraparietal (LIP) area of the parietal cortex respond to cues predicting rewards and penalties of variable size in a manner that depends on the motivational salience of the predicted outcome (strong for both large reward and large penalty) rather than on its value (positive for large reward and negative for large penalty). They considered this finding to suggest that the LIP mediates the capture of attention by salient events and does not encode value in the service of value-based decision-making. Their results indicated that neurons within the amygdala encoded cue value under circumstances in which LIP neurons exhibited sensitivity to motivational salience. As we have stressed elsewhere (Wasserman & Wasserman, 2016) the inclusion of the amygdala indicates the inclusion of emotion-based factors in the determination of value. This conclusion has been supported by research that demonstrates that amygdala neurons facilitate targeting eye movements (saccades) reliably based on aspects of emotional context, as is necessary for goal-directed and social behavior (Maeda, Kunimatsu, & Hikosaka, 2018).

4.5 Expectancy Theory

Human behavior is generally guided by the anticipation of potential outcomes that are considered to be rewarding (Rademacher et al., 2010). Not all outcomes however, are equally rewarding. As we have all experienced, some outcomes are more rewarding, some less so, and some not rewarding at all. Some outcomes are actually, outright undesirable. This general concept has been embodied in the work around expectancy theory (Eccles et al., 1983). When applied to motivation, the expectancy theory of motivation posits that people are motivated to do something because they think their actions will lead to a highly desired outcome (Redmond, 2009). Essentially, expectancy theory hypothesizes that motivation is dependent upon the perceived association between performance of specific actions and their perceived possibility of obtaining certain outcomes. Part of this theory outlines how individuals modify their behavior based on their calculation regarding the probability that certain actions will achieve specific outcomes.

One way to understand the concept of motivation from a neural network perspective is to utilize the idea of anticipation of reward as the basis of its definition. There are neural network analogs that can be used to represent the intensity of the anticipation associated with a specific outcome and help us understand how the power of the anticipation of a particular outcome (set of stimuli) drives goal-directed behavior. Briefly, when competing choices are available, what you select to do is what you anticipate to bring the highest value reward at the lowest expenditure of effort. Motivation is the summed balance between these two forces. The analog that most network models use to reflect these anticipatory choices is probabilistic reward calculations.

4.6 Probabilistic Reward Calculations and the Human Brain

As we have discussed, people make choices of action based upon the anticipation of both rewards and punishments. One way to describe or understand the anticipatory process is to define it in a manner consistent with probabilistic reward theory. Understanding which choice is the most attractive (motivating) is fairly simple and predictable when the options for response differ on only one dimension. For example, if people are offered a choice between two rewards that differ only in amount, they generally choose the larger, rather than the smaller reward. If offered a choice between two rewards that differ only in waiting time for acquisition, people will likely choose the reward available sooner rather than the one available later, and if offered a choice between two options that differ only in probability, they tend to choose the option that they believe will be more likely available. A complementary set of principles for negative outcomes (e.g., smaller punishments will be chosen over larger ones) also apply. These behavioral tendencies obviously make both economic and evolutionary sense (Green & Myerson, 2004).

Things become more interesting and complex when choice options differ on more than one dimension, and that's where probabilistic reward modeling comes in. For example, what happens when a person has to choose between a smaller reward that is available immediately and a larger reward that is available at a later date? How is the relationship between these variables impacted when the larger, delayed reward is more certain than the smaller, immediately available reward? Does the magnitude of the difference impact the choice? For example, Billy mows the lawn of his next door neighbor, Mr. Johnson. Mr. Johnson is short of cash and needs to go to the bank, but the bank is closed and he has to wait for 2 days. He tells Billy he can give him five dollars today, but if he waits until Monday, he can give him six dollars. What does Billy do? Does this calculation change if the sum of ten dollars is available? Does this change if Mr. Johnson is the forgetful type and there is a 50% chance that he will forget the discussion by Monday? Probabilistic reward modeling treats this series of choices as sort of a multiple regression equation, with each variable receiving a certain weighting (positive or negative). These equations result in one number that represents the strength of the choice; One number that represents how "motivating" that choice is in relation to the other available choices.

There is strong behavioral and physiological evidence that the brain both represents probability distributions, and performs probabilistic inference on a continuous basis (Pouget, Beck, Ma, & Latham, 2013). People, as well as other animals, perform near-optimal probabilistic inference in a wide range of cognitive and physical tasks. This probabilistic inference requires trial-to-trial representation of the uncertainties associated with task variables, retention, and subsequent use of this representation (Orhan & Wa, 2017). Essentially, these models use probability to describe how the human brain deals with uncertainty. The models are used to describe how the brain selects a course of action from amongst a group of actions where the known outcome is in some ways uncertain. Humans are continually bombarded by such choices. For example, should I watch TV now and wait to do my homework project over the weekend? Which television show do I wish to select? What should I have for dinner? Should I apply for this particular job? Should I return a particular phone call? Where should I go on vacation?

Choosing (Choice Behavior) involves the weighing of multiple decision variables, such as usefulness, uncertainty, the amount of time between the behavior and the expected reward, or effort. All of these factors combine to create a subjective relative value for each considered option or potential course of action. This relative value also takes into account prior learning about potential rewards (and punishments) that result from prior actions. In a social context, decisions can also involve strategic thinking about the perceived intentions of others and about the impact of others' behavior on one's own outcome. Valuation is also influenced by different emotions that serve to adaptively regulate choices (Sirigu & Duhamel, 2016).

4.7 Expected Value

One way to understand or investigate anticipation (motivation) is to use the concept of expected value (EV). In probabilistic decision-based modeling, the expected value of a particular choice is calculated, and after the choice has been made, the value of the choice can be updated based upon a temporal difference (TD) prediction error between the EV and the reward magnitude (RM) obtained. The EV is measured as the probability of obtaining a reward multiplied by the reward value placed on having the reward (Rolls, McCabe, & Redoute, 2008). The choice and their respective EVs are retained in memory and serve as stimuli to drive future goal-directed behavior.

4.8 Phases of Reward Calculation

As we have mentioned, reward calculation can be conceptualized as being comprised of three phases. The first phase is one of reward anticipation, that is the motivation and desire for a reward and the second phase is one of reward attainment, which describes the acquisition of the reward. The third phase is reward consumption, which is the liking and utilizing of the reward. Although we have introduced networks relative to the three phases, we will describe their operation relative to motivation in greater substance later.

With respect to reward calculation, people make choices in anticipation of rewards all the time. The choices are mediated by networks (cortico-basal ganglia-thalamo-cortico loop) related to emotional responsivity and cognitive framing. An individual then selects a response based upon a number of variables, including what has worked for us in the past, what has the highest probability of being successful in obtaining what we want, and what we perceive to be rewarding based upon our history, personal and cultural values and ethics, or in other words, our associative learning history, incentive valence and positively valenced emotions. Sometimes it may happen that adaptive responses that worked for us in the past are no longer useful strategies. We then have to recalculate all of the above to determine our motivation to move forward in acquiring the reward. Our reward calculations, as well as both the subsequent emotional and behavioral outcomes have implications for both mental health in general, and therapy efficacy specifically.

4.9 Credit Assignment Problem and a Potential Solution

The understanding that selecting the preferred choice from among a number of available, or potentially available options being how the human brain picks the action it will engage in, only gets us so far as regards motivation. That is because in part, the relationships between various options valuations are usually clear only in retrospect. That is, the analysis had to be conducted, the selection action tried, and a determination of its effectiveness made. Much of what we call motivation is actually a memory of a particular analysis of an event and its result, and the ability of that memory to drive goal-directed behavior in the future. When something good happens, we want to know why it happened, and how to make it happen again. This knowledge, or memory, often happens in the absence of the physical presence of future events themselves. For example, let us suppose that I am a lifelong dog owner, and I am now contemplating a replacement for my recently departed pet. I no longer have a dog, but I do have memories of having a dog, and I am able to use these memories of all the wonderful times I spent playing with my dog in the park to reach a decision to purchase a new puppy. All of the prior decisions and analyses that went into that initial decision have been condensed into a few more wide ranging comprehensive memories that I use to drive goal selection (Luyckx, Spitzer, & Summerfield, 2019). After the aforementioned analyses, I am now motivated to buy a dog.

In addition, many events may precede a reward. How do we know, or decide, which of them caused it? This is a crucial aspect of motivation, because these causal attributions in memory serve as triggers for goal-directed behavior. They are in fact, drivers of motivation. For example, a third-grade child goes to school on a particular day and her mother stops to talk to the teacher on the car pick up line at school. The teacher reports to the mother on a number of things that went well for her daughter in school that day, one of which was that the daughter achieved an A on the spelling test. The mom, obviously thrilled at the report, says to the daughter on the way home, "Honey, I am so proud of you about you getting that A on the spelling test." The probabilistic value of a good grade on the spelling test has been altered by the mother's positive feedback and assigned a higher weight. When the next spelling test occurs, the child will have retained that memory and used it to drive performance on the new test. She is now more motivated than before to do well.

This expectation, that reward will be possible, is known as reward motivation (Murty and Adcock, 2014). Reward motivation hypothetically results in enhanced memory encoding for salient events, even if those events are not explicitly associated with reward. This is because over-inclusive memory encoding should occur only during reward motivation, because any salient event encountered during reward motivation is potentially predictive of reward outcomes. Recent research (Murty and Adcock, 2014) suggests that there are defined neural networks that support this process. Functional magnetic resonance imaging during states of high- or low-reward motivation demonstrated motivation amplified hippocampal activation to, and declarative memory for, expectancy violations. Expectancy violations occur when the actual outcome differentiated in a meaningful way from the expected outcome. Connectivity of the ventral tegmental area (VTA) with medial prefrontal, ventrolateral prefrontal, and visual cortices preceded and predicted this increase in hippocampal sensitivity. These findings demonstrate that reward motivation can enhance hippocampus-dependent memory.

4.10 Equifinality, Multifinality, and Counterfinality

There are several models of how conditions and preferences impact strategies used in motivation. All of these represent strategies employed in relation to the selection by an individual in order to obtain a goal. Equifinality is the principle that a given end state can be reached by different means or mechanisms, whereas multifinality is basically the opposite, suggesting that similar conditions or mechanisms can lead to dissimilar outcomes (Nusslock & Alloy, 2017). The multifinality model also refers to a circumstance wherein a single means is seen as serving more than one goal, thus affording the attainment of several objectives via a single activity. The counter finality effect implies the more a means is perceived as detrimental to an alternative goal, the more it is perceived as instrumental to its focal goal (Schumpe, Bélanger, Dugas, Erb, & Kruglanski, 2018). These concepts are also useful when considering the utility of a network model in relation the construct of motivation and its relationship to the reward recognition network.

The research on these concepts is based on the idea that much of what we understand motivation to be is cognitive (Kruglanski, Chernikova, Babush, Dugas, & Schumpe, 2015). That is because values, goals, wishes, and desires are mentally represented, as are their presumed means of attainment. The basic idea of motivation, and its related activity of planning, refers to the building of relations between specific activities and the desirable states of affairs they are presumed to bring about. In creating such constructions, people plan out the motivational space they intend to navigate, and chart the trajectory that offers the best way to meet their goals. This in effect, creates a "mental map" that contains a representation of the various goals which are salient for people when they are faced with specific tasks or situations. These mental maps also contain the representations of possible means to the goals in question, as well as obstacles that may interfere with the attainment of these goals. The final product is a motivationally relevant mental map which consists of interlocking configurations of goals and means, creating conceptual network individuals are contemplating and taking into account when they are making their choices and carrying out their actions (Schumpe et al., 2018). The multifinality configuration refers to a situation wherein a single means is seen as serving more than one goal, thus affording the attainment of several objectives via a single activity. This view is the one that closely conforms to the idea that motivation is a trait that manifests itself in a multiplicity of situations and can be reliably measured across time and task. The multifinality configuration maximizes value that accumulates across the different goals.

In contrast to the multifinality configuration, the idea of equifinality depicts a situation wherein each of a different means leads to a single goal. This implies the need to exercise choice between the different means; it also extends the possibility of substituting, if need be, each of the means for any of the others. For instance, if a given means failed to deliver progress, a different means to the same goal could be taken instead, thus preserving the expectancy that the goal in question will be attained after all. This also corresponds to what we understand as a trait definition of motivation in that the individual would be goal driven and continue to substitute means until the goal was obtained.

Finally, the counterfinality configuration posits a pattern of goals-means relations wherein a means is seen to serve a given focal goal, that is at the same time believed to undermine another goal. This suggests that the selection of certain activities will enhance the value of a specific goal, while at the same time decrease the value of several others.

The multifinality configuration offers enhanced value derived through the attainment of multiple goals through a single activity. As we have seen, however, such enhancement comes at a price, in the form of reduced expectancy of goal attainment mediated by the dilution effect. The equifinality configuration affords increased overall expectancy of goal attainment while diluting the specific expectancy via any of the several means attached to a given goal. Finally, the counterfinality configuration enhances the expectancy that a means which undermines a different goal is particularly likely to bring about the attainment of the focal goal it serves.

What is important to remember, is that each of these models is based on the determination of value and the attachment of value to a particular goal or objective. The strength or amount of value placed on a particular outcome would determine the power of that goal to drive behavior and the willingness of the individual to engage in any of these strategies to obtain the outcome. All of these strategies are based on the idea that one goal supersedes all others in perceived value. Once the outcome is selected, it is conceivable that all, or a combination of these strategies will be employed. For example, the individual might try a preferred means of obtaining a given goal and then failing that might default to less frequently preferred strategies. In any event, it is understandable that the choice of one goal decreases the attractiveness of competing goals and decreases their ability to drive behavior. In any of these circumstances, the choices are driven by the perceived relative value of the goals at hand.

4.11 Interaction of Emotions in the Operation of the Reward Recognition Network

There is evidence that points to the fact that individuals do not calculate utilities explicitly or exactly. Rather, people tend to construct preferences based on their experiences (Gottlieb, Weiss, & Chapman, 2007). For example, people overweight small, medium-sized, and moderately large probabilities, and they also exaggerate risks. However, neither of these findings is anticipated by prospect theory or experience-based decision research. This suggests that people's experiences of events leaks into decisions, even when risk information is explicitly provided (Kusev & van Schaik, 2011). As a result, choices depend strongly on emotionally filtered context, the type of options and the degree of affect associated with these options, and the nature of the presentation of the available options in the decision-making situation. In addition, both value and the probability of an outcome are assessed in a nonlinear fashion with higher values having decreasing marginal gains, and losses being valued greater than gains. In general, low probabilities are overweighted, and high probabilities are underweighted (Kahneman & Tversky, 1979). As we might speculate, emotions play a significant role in these weightings.

There are even models which have the affective regulation networks calculating their own probability weightings, and then interfacing with the reward network to produce a combined weighting. This dual system model (Mukherjee, 2010) incorporates (a) individual differences in disposition to rational versus emotional decision-making, (b) the affective nature of outcomes and, (c) different task constructs within its framework.

The essential takeaway for the practicing clinician is that both emotional states and traits impact reward calculations, and the behavioral choices that result from them. In addition, experiences affect mood, which in turn affects the interpretation and predictive weighting of future experiences. This relationship appears to be governed by two specific principles. First, mood depends on how recent reward outcomes differ from expectations. Second, mood biases the way we perceive outcomes (e.g., rewards), and this bias affects learning about those outcomes. This two-way interaction serves to mitigate inefficiencies in the application of reinforcement learning to real-world problems. In this model mood represents the overall momentum of recent outcomes, and its biasing influence on the perception of outcomes "corrects" learning to account for environmental dependencies. This results in potential dysfunction of adaptive behaviors that have the potential to contribute to the symptoms of mood disorders (Eldar, Rutledge, Dolan, & Niv, 2015).

This makes these reward processes critical targets for the therapeutic process as the new, healthier choices we wish our clients to make are dependent on the outcomes of these selection processes. In addition, their assessment of the success of the experiences they have while they are in treatment and attempting the adaptive behaviors and cognitions are crucial to the therapeutic process.

4.12 Core Brain Dimensions and Mental Health

The National Institute of Mental Health (NIMH) recently launched the Research Domain Criteria (RDoC) initiative (Insel, 2013). This initiative is utilizing five major domains of human functioning. These domains are designed around emotion, cognition, motivation, and social behavior. Within each domain are behavioral elements, processes, mechanisms, and responses, called constructs that comprise different aspects of the overall range of functions. Of importance, (1) the constructs are studied along a span of functioning from normal to abnormal, and (2) with the understanding that each is part of an environmental and neurodevelopmental process, and therefore studied within that context. This initiative encourages the development of new ways of diagnosing disorders of mental health and neurobiologically based disorders based on core brain-behavior dimensions. Rather than work based on behavioral clusters/definitions, RDoC begins with our current understanding of brain-behavior dimensions and aims to link these dimensions to specific symptoms. We will review this initiative and its implications for the process of therapy later. For now, it is important to note that network models work well within this initiative. Consistent with the premise of this book, one stated goal of RDoC is to identify pathophysiological mechanisms that cut across, or are common to, multiple disorders of mental health. Identifying these mechanisms that underlie trans-diagnostic symptom clusters can help break down the behaviorally arbitrary distinctions between categorically defined mental health disorders and account for comorbidity among current DSM diagnostic categories (Nusslock & Alloy, 2017). For example, deficits in threat processing, executive control, and working memory are common to multiple psychiatric conditions. Recent studies into autism have collectively found reduced neural activity in the reward center, specifically the ventral striatum, for both monetary and social rewards, with lower responses to social rewards (Bookheimer, 2010). It makes sense then, and is a primary tenet of this book, to assume a continuum of reinforcement values occurs, and occurs across contexts for neuro-typical brains. By extension then, we must again evaluate the construct of motivation as a unitary event under any given set of circumstances.

4.13 Gating

Gating describes neurological processes of filtering out redundant or unnecessary stimuli in the brain from all possible environmental stimuli. Essentially, gating is the process which modulates input into the brain and insures that the system is not overloaded. This is a crucial management process of the brain because at any one point during the day there is more information coming into the brain than can be effectively processed. Humans need a way to parse that information down to critical elements to which to attend. This parsing is not a passive process, because the human brain actively selects the information to which it will attend based upon a number of variables. Among these variables are prior knowledge, past history of reinforcement and interest.

Gating, which depends upon contribution of the reward system to the allocation of working memory to specific stimuli, involves multiple brain systems operating in concert (McGinty et al., 2011). Learning, which occurs when certain stimuli are selected from the environment to be attended to therefore, is not a passive acceptance of prepackaged knowledge which exists, but involves learners (clients) actively engaging with the material and selecting from the material elements that are meaningful to them in a purposeful and directed way. What is gated, and what is not, is entirely dependent on the individual doing the gating, and the result is by no means predictable by those individuals seeking to impart the knowledge. It is easy to observe gating in action; Simply find a teenager and try to explain something to them for which they have no interest.

4.14 Role of Reward Recognition in the Gating Network

What gets gated, or selected for action, is highly dependent on the history of reinforcement associated with the action. In essence, the higher the probability of a perceived reinforcement, the more likely it is that the stimuli associated with that reinforcement will be gated to attention. In support of this fact, there is emerging research concerning the integration of the reward recognition network with the gating system. In the gating system "reward is a central component for driving incentive-based learning, appropriate responses to stimuli, and the development of goal-directed behaviors" (Haber & Knutson, 2010, p. 4).

There is substantial agreement concerning the cortical and subcortical structural network components for complex, goal-directed human behavior. Specifically, Koziol and Budding (2009) acknowledged the sub thalamic nucleus and ventral pallidum, the subiculum and related hippocampal areas, the lateral habenula, the mesopontine rostromedial tegmental nucleus, the extended amygdala, the bed nucleus of the stria terminals, and the hypothalamus. As is true of other networks, the reward network is not a fixed system. Koziol and Budding conclude by stating "one consistent point that became apparent was that brain regions cannot be simply labeled as either contributing, or not contributing, to motivated behavior; rather, it's necessary to consider the specific circumstances under which the region is being engaged" (p. 356). Hart, Leung and Balleine (2014) point out that "considerable evidence suggests that distinct neural processes mediate the acquisition and performance of goal-directed instrumental actions. Whereas a cortical-dorsomedial striatal circuit appears critical for the acquisition of goal-directed actions, a cortical-ventral striatal circuit appears to mediate instrumental performance, particularly the motivational control of performance" (p. 104). This essentially means that, as expected, automatized behaviors and emotional responses have separate components of the reward recognition network associated with them.

There are other subcortical structures that play a significant role in both gating and reward recognition. One of these is the pedunculopontine nucleus (PPN) (also referred to as pedunculopontine tegmental nucleus, PPTN or PPTg) which is located in the brainstem, to the rear of the substantia nigra and next to the superior cerebellar peduncle. The PPN is historically identified as one of the main components of the reticular activating system (Garcia-Rill, 1991). The PPN projects to a wide variety of cortical and subcortical systems. The PPN plays a significant role in gating both sensorimotor- and reward-related behavior (Diederich & Koch, 2005). Similarly, the nucleus accumbens (NAcc) has been identified as critical in the control of goal-directed behavior. Taha and Fields (2006) found that a subset of NAcc neurons demonstrated a long-lasting inhibition in firing rate, whose onset preceded initiation of goal-directed sequences of behavior, and terminates at the conclusion of the sequence. This firing pattern suggested that, when active, these neurons inhibited goal-directed behaviors and that, when inhibited, these neurons permissively gated those behaviors.

Other cortical structures such as the caudate nucleus are active when learning relationships between stimuli and responses or categories. Seger and Cinotta (2005) found that activity associated with successful learning was localized in the body and tail of the caudate and putamen. Hippocampal activity was associated with receiving positive feedback, but not with correct classification. Successful learning correlated positively with activity in the body and tail of the caudate nucleus, and negatively with activity in the hippocampus.

4.15 Motivation and Gating

One way therefore, to understand the impact of motivation, is to conceptualize gating and its related properties as the neural network underpinning of motivation's cognitive and emotional processing components. While most behavioral learning models conceptualize that reinforcement makes a specific action more likely, the neural network model of motivation emphasizes that reward (value) makes a response to a certain stimulus more likely (Werner, 1994). While gating represents the process around the selection of actions, motivation represents the analysis and culmination (summary) of all the probabilistic reward valuations related to a specific goal. Motivation represents a state of readiness, or action potential, that is stored in long-term memory based upon these summaries. In the case of a newly experienced stimulus, pattern matching allows for these potentials, which have been computed before in relation to similar task to be associated with the new task. These action potentials have been engaged so many times, that in relation to specific tasks, they become highly automated.

This gating-based approach would is based on the use of mental representations of reward calculations, stored in long-term memory, that estimate the distributions of probabilities generated by observing certain events, in particular contexts. There are obviously many types of such events that can be groups together in schemata-based classifications. This would allow for certain classes of events (academics, sports games) that contain specific stimuli to be considered equally motivating. The probabilities that are measured are typically either the probability of observing a certain state, or the probability of observing particular transitions between states, or the probability of observing a particular state after having observed a given state (Oudeyer & Kaplan, 2009). The automated store representations would represent the potential for selection of a course of action. This stored selection bias would represent intrinsic motivation.

It is not clear from the extant literature whether these representations would represent only an analysis of value or would include the other critical variable to the calculation of motivation that is the analysis of the probability that the action would be successful in obtaining the goal. This second major factor in intrinsic motivation is based on assessment of competence that an individual has for achieving self-determined results or goals. Included herein is the concept of difficulty associated with obtaining the selected outcome. It is related to the properties of the achievement process, rather than the meaning of the particular goal being achieved (Oudeyer & Kaplan, 2009). It is unclear at the current time if these mental representations are combined or are stored separately from value considerations. It is likely that both possibilities are present. While in some cases, competence-based and knowledge-based models of intrinsic motivation might be somewhat equivalent in the determination of the selection of outcome, they often produce very different behaviors. For the most part, the capacity to predict what happens in a situation is only weakly associated to the capacity to impact a situation in order to achieve a given self-determined goal.

For example, let's assume that Bill likes a specific type of car and has always wanted to buy one. Let's also assume that Bill has decided that the car would absorb too much of his income. It would be too difficult to maintain. Having thought about this many times it is hard to see how both value and probability of success would not be automated. Now let's assume that Bill gets a promotion and a raise. Many of the obstacles no longer exist. The probability of obtaining equation has to be adjusted. This situation would then represent a circumstance where the value calculation (I still want this) would occur before a new and separate probability of obtaining calculation.

Finally, it is possible that there exist mental representations of the combined analysis (value and effort) where the preferred selection represents neither the value choice nor the effort choice but a compromise between the two. Let's suppose that Bill recognizes that if he worked two nights a week at a second job based at home he would be able to make the money necessary to obtain his second choice car. It wouldn't be perfect, but it would be far more preferable to what he was driving now.

4.16 Attention-Gated Reinforcement Learning (AGREL)

There has been some work attempting to integrate probabilistic reinforcement and the gating of attention as it relates to choice and goal directedness. The attention-gated reinforcement learning model is one of these attempts (Roelfsema & van Ooyen, 2005). This model incorporates two factors that modify synaptic plasticity and lead to a response being gated:

1. A reinforcement signal that is homogeneous across the network and depends on the amount of reward obtained after a trial and,
2. An attentional feedback signal from the output layer that limits plasticity to those units at earlier processing levels that are crucial for the stimulus-response mapping.

The first factor is a global reward-related signal. This signal reaches all relevant synapses and is presumably implemented in the brain by the release of neuromodulators. In AGREL, the first factor represents the difference between the amount of reward that is expected, and the amount that is actually obtained.

The second factor is a site-specific effect due to the feedback of neuronal activity, which assigns credit to sensory neurons that play a critical role in the selection of an action. In AGREL a brain site-specific factor is used to represent the assignment credit to hidden units that make up a network that is responsible for the selected/preferred action. This is accomplished by a feedback signal from the winning output unit to the units that made it win. In AGREL, the winning motor program feeds its activity back to all elements of the selected/recruited network. These connections between feedforward and feedback areas are reciprocal. As a result, if network components have strong feedforward they usually also receive strong feedback from these same network elements. The consequence of this reciprocity is that neurons that provide the strongest excitation to a particular motor program also receive the strongest feedback, and are then more likely to be utilized when a target goal (or highly similar circumstance) is identified.

As we have stated elsewhere, it is clear that learning gates attention and that the value attributed to that learning gates attention (Wasserman & Wasserman, 2015). It is also clear that the history of success or failure of that directed attention is stored in working memory to be called upon in future circumstances. It is therefore possible to conceptualize these stored memories regarding the value and probability of success as the neural network property of motivation.

4.17 Summary

A chapter summary here poses a difficult pursuit as a perusal of the subchapters contained herein highlights the complexities of understanding motivation within a neural network model. When considering this construct, what should be clear from the aforementioned chapter, is that the process is complex and multi-determined, requiring the inclusion of internal and external variables, consideration of how one develops a value for a particular event or stimulus, and how many factors must be considered in order to motivate the person to action. We have attempted to focus on the anticipation, attainment, valuation, and consummatory aspects of reward in this chapter as it defines motivation and neural networks. As we have pointed out, to understand motivation, you have to understand reward. We have chosen to frame the concept of reward within a valuation or neuroeconomic model. This allows for the potential of concepts such as motivation to be quantified as well as qualified. While this quantification process is still in its infancy, the goal would of course, be to be able to correlate the methods with clinical findings such as neuropsychological testings and observable or self report measures.

We have attempted to address how one attends to, conceptualizes and values a particular reward, and tie it to a neural network base, in this particular case, with the reward network as the focus, to address the development of internal and external motivations. As we can see from the large number of network functions involved, motivation is the result of a highly interactive network system. It is important to remember that these networks are not permanent. They are recruited in a task dependent manner with each component playing a specific role.

References

Berridge, K., & Robinson, T. (1998). What is the role of dopamine in reward: hedonic impact, reward learning, or incentive salience? *Brain Research: Brain Research Review, 28*, 309–369. https://doi.org/10.1016/s0165-0173(98)00019-8.

Bookheimer, A. A.-V. (2010). Reward processing in autism. *Autism Research, 3*, 53–67.

Browne, C., Godino, A., Salery, M., & Nestler, E. (2020). *Epigenetic mechanisms of opioid addiction biological psychiatry, 87*(1), 22–33. https://doi.org/10.1016/j.biopsych.2019.06.027.

Diederich, K., & Koch, M. (2005). Role of the pedunculopontine tegmental nucleus in sensorimotor gating and reward-related behavior in rats. *Psychopharmacology, 179*(2), 402–408.

Eccles, J., Adler, T. F., Futterman, R., Goff, S., Kaczala, C. M., Meece, J., & Midgley, C. (1983). Expectancies, values and academic behaviors. In J. Spense (Ed.), *Achievement and achievement motives*. San Francisco: W. H. Freeman.

Eldar, E., Rutledge, R., Dolan, R., & Niv, Y. (2015). Mood as representation of momentum. *Trends in Cognitive Neuroscience, 20*(1), 15–24. https://doi.org/10.1016/j.tics.2015.07.010.

Garcia-Rill, E. (1991). The pedunculopontine nucleus. *Progress in Neurobiology, 36*(5), 363–389.

Gottlieb, D., Weiss, T., & Chapman, G. (2007). The format in which uncertainty information is presented affects decision biases. *Psychological Science, 18*(3), 240–246.

Green, L., & Myerson, J. (2004). A discounting framework for choice with delayed and probabilistic rewards. *Psychological Bulletin, 130*(5), 769–792. https://doi.org/10.1037/0033-2909.130.5.769.

Haber, S., & Knutson, B. (2010). The reward circuit: Linking primate anatomy and human imagery. *Neuropshycopharmacology, 35*(1), 4–26.

Hart, G., Leung, B. K., & Balleine, B. W. (2014). Dorsal and ventral streams: the distinct role of striatal subregions in the acquisition and performance of goal-directed actions. *Neurobiology of learning and memory, 108*, 104–118. https://doi.org/10.1016/j.nlm.2013.11.003.

Insel, T. (2013, April 29). *Directors Blog: Transforming diagnosis*. National Institute of Mental Health. Retrieved from http://www.nimh.nih.gov/about/director/2013/transforming-diagnosis.shtml.

Kahneman, D., & Tversky, A. (1979). Prospect theory: An analysis of decision under risk. *Econometrica, 47*, 263–291.

Kal, B., Case, J., Freed, R., Stern, E., & Gabbay, V. (2017). Neural correlates of RDoC reward constructs in adolescents with diverse psychiatric symptoms: A Reward Flanker Task pilot study. *J Affect Disord, 216*, 36–45. https://doi.org/10.1016/j.jad.2016.11.042.

Kelley, A., & Berridge, K. (2002). The neuroscience of natural rewards: Relevance to addiction. *The Journal of Neuroscience, 22*(9), 3306–3311.

Koziol, L., & Budding, D. (2009). Subcortical structures and cognition springer international publishing. ISBN 978-0-387-84868-6.

Kruglanski, A., Chernikova, M., Babush, M., Dugas, M., & Schumpe, B. M. (2015). The architecture of goal systems: Multifinality, equifinality, and counterfinality in means—End relations. In A. Elliot (Ed.), *Advances in motivation science* (Vol. 2, pp. 69–98). Philadephia: Elsevier, Academic Press.

Kusev, P., & van Schaik, P. (2011). Preferences under risk: content-dependent behavior and psychological. *Frontiers in Psychology, 2*, 269. https://doi.org/10.3389/fpsyg.2011.00269.

Leathers, M., & Olsen, C. (2017). In monkeys making value-based decisions, amygdala neurons are sensitive to cue value as distinct from cue salience. *Journal of Neurophysiology, 117*(4), 1499–1511. https://doi.org/10.1152/jn.00564.2016.

Leathers, M., & Olson, C. (2012). In monkeys making value-based decisions, LIP neurons encode cue salience and not action value. *Science, 338*(6103), 132–135.

Luyckx, F. N., Spitzer, B., & Summerfield, C. (2019). Neural structure mapping in human probabilistic reward learning. *eLife, 8*, e42816. https://doi.org/10.7554/eLife.42816.

Maeda, K., Kunimatsu, J., & Hikosaka, O. (2018). Amygdala activity for the modulation of goal-directed behavior in emotional contexts. *PLoS Biology, 16*(6), e2005339. https://doi.org/10.1371/journal.pbio.2005339. eCollection 2018 Jun.

McGinty, V., Hayden, B., Heilbronner, S., Dumont, E., Graves, S., Mirrione, M., et al. (2011). Emerging, reemerging, and forgotten brain areas of the reward circuit: Notes from the 2010 motivational and neural networks conference. *Behavioural Brain Research, 225*, 348–357. https://doi.org/10.1016/j.bbr.2011.07.036. Retrieved from National Institute of Health.

Mukherjee, K. (2010). A dual system model of preferences under risk. *Pyschological Review, 117*, 243–255. https://doi.org/10.1037/a0017884.

Murty, V., & Adcock, R. (2014). Enriched encoding: reward motivation organizes cortical networks for hippocampal detection of unexpected events. *Cerebral Cortex, 24*(8), 2160–2168. https://doi.org/10.1093/cercor/bht063.

Nestler, E. (2014). Epigenetic mechanisms of drug addiction. *Neuropharmacology, 76*, 259–268.

Nusslock, R., & Alloy, L. (2017). Reward processing and mood-related symptoms: An RDoC and reward processing and mood-related symptoms. *Journal of Affective Disorders, 216*, 3–16. https://doi.org/10.1016/j.jad.2017.02.001.

Orhan, A., & Wa, W. (2017). Efficient probabilistic inference in generic neural networks trained with non-probabilistic feedback. *Nature Communications, 8*(1), 138. https://doi.org/10.1038/s41467-017-00181-8.

Oudeyer, P., & Kaplan, F. (2009). What is intrinsic motivation? A typology of computational approaches. *Frontiers in Neurorobotics, 1*, 16. https://doi.org/10.3389/neuro.12.006.2007.

Pochon, J., Levy, R., Fossati, P., Lehericy, S., Poline, J., Pillon, B., et al. (2002). The neural system that bridges reward and cognition in humans: An fMRI study. *PNAS, 99*(8), 5669–5674. https://doi.org/10.1073/pnas.082111099.

Pouget, A., Beck, J., Ma, W., & Latham, P. (2013). Probabilistic brains: Knowns and unknowns. *Nature Neuroscience, 16*(9), 1170–1178. https://doi.org/10.1038/nn.3495.

Rademacher, L., Krach, S., Kohls, F., Irmak, A., Gründera, G., & Spreckelmeyera, K. (2010). Dissociation of neural networks for anticipation and consumption of monetary and social rewards. *NeuroImage, 49*(4), 3276–s3265. https://doi.org/10.1016/j.neuroimage.2009.10.089.

Ranganath, C. (2010). A unified framework for the functional organization of the medial temporal lobes and the phenomenology of episodic memory. *Hippocampus, 20*, 1263–1290.

Redmond, B. (2009). Lesson 4: Expectancy theory: Is there a link between my effort and what I want?. *Academic Leadership*. Retrieved from:http://www.academicleadership.org/empirical_research/466_printer.shtml.

Roelfsema, P., & van Ooyen, A. (2005). Attention-gated reinforcement learning of internal. *Neural Computation, 17*, 2176–2214.

Rolls, E., McCabe, C., & Redoute, J. (2008). Expected value, reward outcome, and temporal difference error representations in a probabilistic decision task. *Cerebral Cortex, 18*, 652–663. https://doi.org/10.1093/cercor/bhm097.

Schultz, W. (2015). Neuronal reward and decision signals: From theories to data. *Physiological Reviews, 95*(3), 853–951.

Schumpe, B., Bélanger, J., Dugas, M., Erb, H., & Kruglanski, A. (2018). Counterfinality: On the increased perceived instrumentality of means to a goal. *Frontiers in Psychology, 9*, 1052. https://doi.org/10.3389/fpsyg.2018.01052.

Sirigu, S., & Duhamel, J. (2016). Reward and decision processes in the brains of humans and nonhuman primates. *Dialogues in Clinical Neuroscience, 18*(1), 45–53.

Seger, C. A., & Cincotta, C. M. (2005). The roles of the caudate nucleus in human classification learning. *The Journal of neuroscience : the official journal of the Society for Neuroscience, 25*(11), 2941–2951. https://doi.org/10.1523/JNEUROSCI.3401-04.2005.

Taha, S. A., & Fields, H. L. (2006). Inhibitions of nucleus accumbens neurons encode a gating signal for reward-directed behavior. *The Journal of neuroscience : the official journal of the Society for Neuroscience, 26*(1), 217–222. https://doi.org/10.1523/JNEUROSCI.3227-05.2006.

Wasserman, T., & Wasserman, L. (2015). The misnomer of attention deficit hyperactivity disorder. *Journal of Applied Neuropsychology, 4*(2), 116–122. https://doi.org/10.1080/21622965.2015.1005487.

Wasserman, T., & Wasserman, L. (2016). *Depathologizing psychopathology*. New York: Springer.

Wasserman, T., & Wasserman, L. (2017). *Neurocognitive learning therapy; theory and practice*. New York: Springer.

Werner, G. (1994). Using second order neural connections for motivation of behavioral choices. In P. Husbands, J. Meyer, & S. Wilson (Eds.), *From animals to animals 3: Proceedings of the third international conference* (pp. 155–162). Cambridge: MIT Press.

Yi, W., Mei, S., Zhang, M., & Zheng, Y. (2020). Decomposing the effort paradox in reward processing: Time matters. *Neuropsychologia, 137*, 107311. https://doi.org/10.1016/j.neuropsychologia.2019.107311.

Zhang, Y., Wang, Z., Li, Q., Liu, X., & Zhen, Y. (2017). Temporal dynamic of reward anticipation in the human brain. *Biological Psychology, 128*, 89–97.

Chapter 5
Motivation as Goal-Directed Behavior: The Effect of Decision-Making

People are often faced with complex, uncertain situations that require decisive actions in order to pursue short- or long-term goals. Learning to choose adaptively between different behavioral options in order to reach these goals is a ubiquitous task in life, for people of all ages. The actual achievement of goals can be rewarding. The process of achieving goals is also important. Monitoring of both the ongoing action-based processes and the outcomes of these behavioral options is necessary for goal attainment. Adaptive behavior requires interactions between processes that monitor action–outcome relations and mechanisms that evaluate these relations with respect to goal significance in order to modify future actions based on these evaluations (Eppinger, Hämmerer, & Li, 2011). These choices reach across the life spectrum and range from the process entailed in reaching for a desired object in a potentially unsafe area, such as a desired toy next to a large dog or retrieving a football held by the other team, to deciding between jobs, one with potentially better long-term career implications versus one offering more initial pay, or to gambling in a casino. How we make those choices between options has been studied under the general term of decision-making.

5.1 The Neurophysiology of Decision-Making

Where and how in the brain are the estimates of expected reward represented and updated by the animal's experience? There is converging evidence from a number of recent studies, which suggest that many of these computations are carried out in multiple interconnected regions in the frontal cortex and basal ganglia (Lee, Seo, & Jung, 2012). Full discussions of the neural networks and their development and involvement regarding these areas are presented in adjoining chapters. We are turning our attention here specifically to the network as it impacts probabilistic valuation.

T. Wasserman, L. Wasserman, *Motivation, Effort, and the Neural Network Model*, Neural Network Model: Applications and Implications,
https://doi.org/10.1007/978-3-030-58724-6_5

5.2 The Anterior Cingulate Cortex (ACC) and Effort-Based Valuation

If a person is faced with a choice between two courses of immediate action, one of which leads to a larger reward than the other, then it is simple to figure out which is more valuable and therefore which they should choose. As we have said, up until now that was the basis for understanding the value-based model. That particular circumstance is more the exception than the rule. Often there are mitigating circumstances. For example, if the same choice is presented except that now the larger reward is only obtained after a period of time has elapsed or a larger amount of effort has been expended, then the optimal decision is no longer so clear. This decrease of the value of a reward by the cost incurred to achieve it is known as discounting and has been shown consistently to influence the way in which animals and humans make choices (Walton, Rudebeck, Bannerman, & Rushworth, 2007).

As we have indicated, people's preferences for one course of action over another reflect not just reward expectations but also the cost in terms of effort that must be invested in pursuing the course of action. Research has demonstrated that cue-locked activity in the ventral striatum and midbrain reflected the net (final) value of the course of action, signaling the expected amount of reward discounted by the amount of effort to be invested. Activity in ACC also reflects the interaction of both expected reward and effort costs. Posterior orbitofrontal and insular activity, however, only reflected the expected reward magnitude. The ventral striatum and anterior cingulate cortex may be the substrate of effort-based cost–benefit valuation in humans (Croxson, Walton, O'Reilly, Behrens, & Rushworth, 2009).

There is also evidence that the ACC working in conjunction with the dorsal striatum (dorsal putamen) signal the anticipation of effort independently of the prospect of winning or losing. This research indicated that activity in ventral striatum (ventral putamen) was greater for better-than-expected outcomes compared with worse-than-expected outcomes, an effect attenuated in the context of having exerted greater effort. This research demonstrated that neural representations of anticipated actions are sensitive to the expected demands, but not to the expected value of their consequence, whereas representations of outcome value are discounted by exertion, commensurate with an integration of cost and benefit so as to approximate net value (Kurniawan, Guitart-Masip, Dayan, & Dolan, 2013).

5.3 Behavioral Economics, Cost and Valuation

Behavioral economic modeling is a good way to understand neural network valuation modeling. Decision-making consists of choosing among available options on the basis of a valuation of both their potential costs and benefits. Most theoretical models of decision-making in behavioral economics, psychology, and computer science propose that the desirability of outcomes expected from alternative options can be quantified by utility functions. These utility functions allow a decision-maker to assign subjective values to each option under consideration by weighting the likely benefits and costs resulting from an action and to select the one with the highest subjective value. Research has demonstrated that the human brain uses distinct valuation subsystems for different types of costs, reflecting in opposite fashion delayed reward and future energetic expenses. The ventral striatum and the ventromedial prefrontal cortex represent the increasing subjective value of delayed rewards, whereas a distinct network, composed of the anterior cingulate cortex and the anterior insula, represent the decreasing value of the effortful option, coding the expected expense of energy. Together, these data demonstrate that the valuation processes underlying different types of costs can be parsed at the neural network level (Prevost, Pessiglione, Metereau, Clery-Melin, & Dreher, 2010).

Neuropsychological studies have demonstrated that parts of the frontal lobe are integral for goal-directed action selection, strategy-implementation and social behavior, all of which are essential components of optimal decision-making (Bechara & Damasio, 2000). There is research that suggests that lesions of the anterior cingulate cortex caused individuals to become less willing to invest effort for reward. These same individuals showed no change when having to tolerate delays. Other research has identified the sulcal region of the anterior cingulate cortex as essential for dynamically integrating over time the recent history of choices and outcomes. Patients with damage to parts of prefrontal cortex can simultaneously exhibit prolonged deliberation about choices accompanied by subsequent irresponsible, risky behavior (Manes et al., 2002). At the same time, studies have shown that the exact same lesions can cause symptoms of apathy and indifference as well as poor impulse control (Levy & Dubois, 2006).

There are, on occasion social costs involved in choice selection. For example, choosing a particular course of social action may also involve additional work and expense of effort such as gathering important information about the people you are potentially interacting with. Evaluating social information when deciding whether to respond has been demonstrated to be a function of the anterior cingulate gyrus. Taken as a whole, this research indicates that there are dissociable pathways in the frontal lobe for managing different types of response cost and for gathering social information.

So, as we can see the neural network properties of the probabilistic valuation system that adds and discounts valuation are clearly elucidated.

5.4 Decision-Making

The primary purpose of the field of decision neuroscience is to understand the neural network properties and mechanisms underlying human decision-making and reward valuation. While it is quite clear that all choice preferences are subjective, many studies have focused on objective properties of decision options, such as reward magnitude or probability, when discussing how decision-making processes occur (Peters & Buchel, 2009). Subjective choice variables have been extensively studied as well. These include the domains of probabilistic and intertemporal decision-making delay discounting (DD) and probability discounting (PD). That is, how long until the reward can be acquired, and how likely is it. This refers to the phenomena that the subjective value of rewards declines in a hyperbolic manner with both increasing delay-to-reward variables and with decreasing reward probability (Green & Myerson, 2004). These factors become more complex as when the choice options vary across more than one variable, such as how long until one could receive the reward *and* how likely is it, or when considering the amount of reward (large vs. small) *and* when it would be attainable (immediate vs. delayed) *and* how probable attainment is. Green and Myerson (2004) highlight that this is not a single process account.

5.5 Reinforcement Learning Theories of Decision-Making

In order to understand motivated behavior we must first understand how people choose between various options, and what informs and directs these choices. One way to understand the interplay of choice and human brain function is to understand the concept of reinforcement learning. Reinforcement learning is a critical component in neural network models of learning, and by extension motivation. It is also a vital component the newly emerging areas of neuroeconomics and decision neuroscience which we will review below. Reinforcement learning is an ongoing adaptive process wherein an individual utilizes previous experience to inform and improve the outcomes of future choices.

In reinforcement learning models, actions are chosen according to their value functions, which describe how much future reward is expected from each action. Value functions can be adjusted not only through reward and penalty, but also by the person's knowledge of its current environment (Lee et al., 2012). Reinforcement learning theories describe how a person's experience changes their determination value functions. This in turn, influences the selection from amongst future choices.

5.6 Economic Models of Decision-Making

Economic theories of decision-making focus on how numbers can be attached to alternative actions so that choices can be understood as selecting an action that has the maximum value among all possible actions. These hypothetical quantities are often referred to as utilities and can be applied to all types of behaviors. By definition, behaviors chosen by an organism are those that maximize the organism's utility. These theories are largely agnostic about how these utilities are determined, although they are presumably constrained by evolution and individual experience.

5.7 Neuroeconomics

One newer way that attempts to understand the goal seeking and goal-directed behavior of humans is the study of neuroeconomics. Neuroeconomics combines the study of the neurobiological and computational bases of value (probabilistic reward valuation)-based decision-making. Its goal is to provide a neurologically/biologically based account of human behavior that can be applied in both natural and the social science settings (Rangel, Camerer, & Montague, 2008).

There are five neuroeconomics model type computations required for value-based decision-making. These computations are represented in the figure below (Rangel et al., 2008):

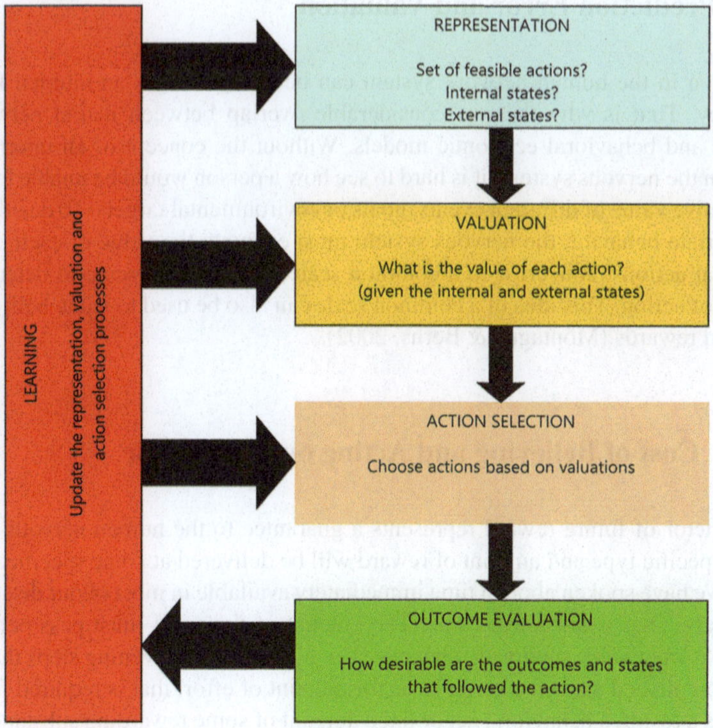

In actuality, this value-based decision-making is pervasive in its implications for human behavior. It occurs whenever a person makes a choice from several alternatives based on the subjective value placed on them. As we have seen, these value-based decisions (probabilistic reward calculations) serve as the basis for network models of goal-directed behavior or motivation. Neuroeconomics is a relatively new field, which analyzes the hypothetical computations that the brain makes in order to make the multiplicity of value-based decisions that occur doing the day.

5.8 Cost

Up until now we have discussed the value added portions of probabilistic reward valuations. We have mentioned that variables such as the amount of effort, the length of time that is required to wait, and other factors that actually serve to decrease the overall valuation of a goal or value. These are termed costs. In order to be able to make informed and successful decisions, it is vital to be able to evaluate whether the expected benefits of a course of action make it worth tolerating the costs incurred to obtain them (Walton et al., 2007).

5.9 Prediction Error and Valuation

Valuation in the human network system can be thought of as an internal form of currency. That is why there is considerable overlap between neural networking models and behavioral economic models. Without the concept of an internal currency in the nervous system, it is hard to see how a person would be unable to assess the relative value of different events, goals or environmental targets. To decide on an appropriate behavior, the nervous system must estimate the value of each of these potential actions, convert it to a common scale, and use this scale to determine a course of action. This idea of a common scale can also be used to value both predictors and rewards (Montague & Berns, 2002).

5.10 Cost of Believing and Acting on a Predictor

A predictor of future reward represents a guarantee to the human nervous system that a specific type and amount of reward will be delivered at some specified future time. We have spoken about a time immediately available in most of our discussions until now. That is not always true. The amount of time that must pass before the reward is obtainable obviously changes. The number of intervening steps that must be accomplished also changes as does the amount of effort that is required for each step. As a result, a behavioral act or fixed amount of some rewarding substance does not possess a fixed value to the organism. The valuation of a reward can change dramatically as new, unanticipated information arrives. Suppose you are working in a factory-making clothing. You must make ten items of clothing to get compensated. One day you come to work and after making right items of clothing the supervisor comes over and says you are now getting your payment or, as is far more likely you bring the ten articles of clothing to the supervisor who tells you that the rules have changed and you now need twelve articles of clothing in order to be paid (rewarded). The question that arises is should the decreased value of the reward also cause a decrease in the value of the predictor for that reward?

To value a predictor, a neural system must have a way to compute the predictor's value before the reward that it suggests will be coming actually arrives. One potential area of uncertainty derives from the time interval extending from predictor onset to the expected future time of reward delivery. However, this uncertainty is important because it effects that valuation of the future reward. A prediction must therefore be made. As we have seen human networks have prediction functions built into them. That is because predictions about future reward represent the potential of increased expenditure of time, effort, and resource of the person. Believing and following a predictor with behavioral action, means that processing time is tied up and behavioral resources committed as actions are prepared. As humans possess finite cognitive and behavioral capital choosing a path to follow represents a potentially costly commitment. Therefore not only the goal must be valued. It follows from the above, that there must exist neural signals that provide an ongoing valuation of both predictors, their intermediate steps and the potential future rewards. It also follows that this system applies equally to both anticipated positive and negative outcomes. Finally, it becomes obvious that some of these predictors are in error to a greater or lesser degree. Therefore humans must possess the network capacity to evaluate the impact and significance of this prediction error.

5.11 Things that Discount the Probabilistic Value of Future Goals

Any valuation system for predicting reward must take account of several important principles. For example, any estimate of future reward is not exact. The future reward may have less or greater value when you receive it. Uncertainty increases with time and more uncertainty will accumulate for reward estimates in the distant future than for those in the near future. For example, I can offer to give you $100 dollars for work you do today or promise to pay you $120 over the next year if you let me pay you out. Whether or not this is a good idea is clearly determined by interest rates, the decreasing value of money whether I need the money or not. Or, in another example, I can give you the option to buy furniture today and not pay me for a year and charge you no interest. Many companies use these types of inducements because people view them as getting the use of the money for free.

There is also risk associated with the future time that separates the predictor from future reward; therefore, there must be some discounting of time, because more time means that there is more risk that something could go wrong.

In both instances, uncertainty increases as time passes and the possibility that one's prediction will be in error increases. Research suggests that orbitofrontal (OFS) circuits act to generate a common internal currency (scale) for the valuation of payoffs, losses, and their proxies (predictors of payoffs and losses) (O'Doherty, Rolls, Bowtell, & McGlone, 2001).

5.12 Discounting

Delay discounting can be defined as the cognitive process that allows a person to compare values between the immediate and delayed consumption of a determined outcome, goal, or commodity. Specifically, delay discounting implies that the value of a reward declines with increasing delay. This delay can be due to simply a temporal issue or can be due to a combined effect of several issues such as time, amount of reward, risk, and effort required to obtain the goal. This is represented by the common research finding that humans often sacrifice a large delayed reward in order to receive a smaller but more immediate reward. Such a choice has been labeled impulsivity. The opposite choice, being able to delay action to achieve a higher value reward has been labeled self-control (Johnson & Bickel, 2002).

A related term, temporal discounting refers to the tendency of people to discount rewards as they approach a temporal horizon in the future or the past. It refers to a point in time so distant that the rewards cease to be valuable or to have other additive effects regarding the driving of choice actions. Choices often involve outcomes that occur at different points in time and/or outcomes that are more or less likely to occur. Such choices have been studied under the labels intertemporal choice and risky choice, respectively. Intertemporal and risky choice represent traditional topics in microeconomics and are critical for understanding many aspects of decision-making (Myerson, Green, Hanson, Holt, & Estle, 2003). Findings from this line of research general indicate that amount of reward has the opposite effects on temporal and probability discounting. Specifically, smaller delayed rewards are discounted more steeply than larger delayed rewards, whereas larger (in terms of risk) probabilistic rewards were discounted more steeply than smaller probabilistic rewards.

5.13 Uncertainty

Uncertainty is one of those psychological constructs with multiple definitions but we will define it here as the psychological state in which a decision-maker lacks exact knowledge about what outcome will follow from what choice (Platt & Huettel, 2008). The aspect of uncertainty most commonly considered by both economists and neuroscientists is risk, which references situations with a known distribution of possible outcomes. Estimates of risk as it relates to a specific value reward are referred to as expected value. When mechanisms for dealing with uncertain outcomes fail, as occur in several mental disorders such as conduct disorder, or more specifically problems with gambling or addiction, the results can be catastrophic.

There are problems with expected utility (value) models in that they often fail to describe the complex issues confronted by most people in the real world. A number of issues, some of them we have already mentioned (allocation of effort, time) lead to systematic violations of expected utility models. These factors serve to modify value calculations by decreasing, or to a lesser extent, increasing eventual probability value assessments. Individuals tend to avoid risky options that could result in either a potential loss or a potential gain, even when the option has a positive expected value.

Some parameters are known. For example, most people will reject (not take) risks until the size of the potential gain becomes approximately twice as large as the size of the potential loss. This particular rule is known as loss aversion (Tom, Fox, Trepel, & Poldrack, 2007). Loss aversion may reflect competition between distinct systems for losses and gains or unequal responses within a single system supporting both types of outcomes. Both gains and losses evoke activation in similar regions, including the striatum, midbrain, ventral prefrontal cortex, and anterior cingulate cortex, with activation increasing with potential gain but decreasing with potential loss.

5.14 Effort

Effort refers to the idiosyncratic intensification of mental and/or physical activity done with the intention of achieving some goal or serving some value (Eisenberger, 1992). It is a process that mediates between how well an organism can potentially perform on some task, and how well they actually perform on that task (Shenhav et al., 2017). This helps explain the phenomena of people failing to be effortful on easy tasks because they are disinterested in the outcome. Effort is the result of motivation. It is not the same as motivation, which is a force that drives behavior by determining both a direction (e.g., goal) and the intensity or vigor with which this direction is pursued (Pessiglione, Vinckier, Bouret, Daunizeau, & Le Bouc, 2017). Effort refers to the intensity or amplitude of behavior, but does not refer to any specific goal although, it does not occur in the absence of a goal or direction.

Effort is a volitional, intentional process, something that people apply. It relates to what people are actively doing, and not to what is passively happening to them. Effort is distinguishable from demand or difficulty: effort corresponds to the intensity of mental or physical work that people exert toward some outcome, whereas demand or difficulty refers to a property of the task itself. Although effort typically tracks demand (with people working harder when the task is more difficult), this relationship breaks down when incentives are too low or when demands are too high (Brehm & Self, 1989).

5.15 Cognitive Effort as a Mediator of Motivation

As we have seen earlier, cognitive effort is often confused, or taken as a stand in for, motivation. At the most basic level, effort references the degree of engagement with demanding tasks. High engagement, representing motivation, may enhance performance by way of attention. Cognitive effort is not motivation, though the effects of increased motivation on performance are definitely mediated by increased effort.

What we now know is that cognitive effort mediates the behavioral or physiological consequences of motivation. A related term, cognitive fatigue, represents decreasing performance and physiological responsiveness to task events over extended time involvement with demanding tasks. It is hypothesized to be partly volitional, since other motivational incentives can counteract fatigue effects (Boksem & Tops, 2008). On the other hand, specific motivational effects can counteract "depletion" effects which occurs when the individual is willing to exert self-control declines with protracted exertion of self-control (Westbrook & Braver, 2015).

The motivation to exert effort for reward is highly subjective and varies considerably across the different domains of behavior. Research has demonstrated that reward devaluation reflective of effort, both cognitive and physical, is subserved by a common neural network of areas, including the dorsomedial and dorsolateral prefrontal cortex, the intraparietal sulcus, and the anterior insula. Activity within these domain-general areas also covaried negatively with reward and positively with effort, suggesting an integration of these parameters within these areas. Additionally, the amygdala appeared to play a unique, domain-specific role in processing the value of rewards associated with cognitive effort (Chong et al., 2017b).

5.16 The Possible Paradox of Effort as a Cost Factor

While most major models in cognitive psychology, neuroscience, and economics, consider effort, be it physical or mental, to be strictly costly. That is, when given a choice, people tend to avoid effort. However, there is emerging evidence that the opposite is also true, and that effort can also add value within a probabilistic valuation model. Some outcomes become more rewarding if we apply more, rather than less effort, and sometimes we select options precisely because they require effort (Inzlicht, Shenhav, & Olivola, 2018). Think about skiing. Many skiers like to challenge themselves by skiing down the more difficult and demanding courses. They often evaluate themselves in comparison to one's abilities or their performance on the "expert" or more demanding courses. This demonstrates that people will work hard to obtain something of value, and that working hard can also make those same things in turn, more valuable. Effort can even be experienced as valuable or rewarding in its own right (Brehm & Self, 1989).

5.17 Effort Is Usually Thought to Decrease Valuation

The idea that effort is costly is supported by many lines of evidence. This idea is based on the indication that the harder something is, the more motivation it takes to do it. As people strive for efficiency, increased effort's cost is greater, and is to be avoided whenever possible. In fact, research demonstrates that increasing effort actually primes adverse physiological and emotional responses (Dreisbach & Fischer, 2012). We are designed to conserve our resources.

Behaviorally, there are well known signs that people often dislike and devalue hard work. Effort, both mental and physical, is typically avoided, and when given tasks that offer equal rewards, but different levels of demand, people usually learn to avoid the more demanding one. In addition, willingness to exert effort usually decreases as a function of the amount of effort already applied (Kool & Botvinick, 2014). It is also clear that effort expenditure does eventually decline with time on task (Blain, Hollard, & Pessiglione, 2016). Another indication that effort is costly comes from the finding that people are often willing to accept fewer rewards to avoid effort (Apps, Grima, Manohar, & Husain, 2015). That is, just as people discount rewards by their associated delays (Olivola & Wang, 2016), they also discount rewards by the amount of cognitive or physical effort required to obtain them (i.e., effort discounting) (Chong et al., 2017a, b).

5.18 Effort Also Adds Value

Social psychology has long recognized the effect of cognitive dissonance and its relationship to effort. This research has consistently demonstrated that the more effort is exerted to obtain things, the more value the said items or achievements are assigned retrospectively (Cooper, 2007). More recent research has provided evidence of effort's added value in the human brain. People receiving rewarding feedback for effortful performance amplify their hemodynamic and electrophysiological signals generated by brain areas sensitive to reward (e.g., subgenual anterior cingulate cortex, caudate, nucleus accumbens, striatum, feedback-related negativity/reward positivity). This is muted or sometimes absent for non-effortful performance (Botvinick, Huffstetler, & McGuire, 2009).

There is also a role for automaticity in the development of effort. Automaticity has a value additive function. If high effort is consistently paired with high reward, this can form a conditioned association, with effort itself taking on the status of a secondary reinforcer (Eisenberger, 1992).

It is clear that effort can either raise or lower value. What it does is dependent on the life course of the individual and the experiences that they have had. Effort, like many other value mediators, is interpreted within the context in which it is learned.

References

Apps, M., Grima, L., Manohar, S., & Husain, M. (2015). The role of cognitive effort in subjective reward devaluation and risky decision-making. *Science Reports, 5*, 16880. https://doi.org/10.1038/srep16880.

Bechara, A. D., & Damasio, A. (2000). Emotion, decision making and the orbitofrontal cortex. *Cerebral Cortex March, 10*(3), 295–307.

Blain, B., Hollard, G., & Pessiglione, M. (2016). Neural mechanisms underlying the impact of daylong cognitive work on economic decisions. *Proceedings of the National Academy of Science, 113*, 6967–6972.

Boksem, M., & Tops, M. (2008). Mental fatigue: Costs and benefits. *Brain Research Reviews, 59*, 125–139. https://doi.org/10.1016/j.brainresrev.2008.07.001.

Botvinick, M., Huffstetler, S., & McGuire, J. (2009). Effort discounting in human nucleus accumbens. *Cognition, Affect and Behavioral Neuroscience, 9*, 16–27.

Brehm, J., & Self, E. (1989). The intensity of motivation. *Annual Review of Psychology, 400*, 109–131.

Chong, T., Apps, M., Giehl, K., Sillence, A., Grima, L. L., & Husain, M. (2017a). Neurocomputational mechanisms underlying subjective valuation of effort. *PLoS Biology, 15*, 1–28.

Chong, T., Apps, M., Giehl, K., Sillence, L. A., Grima, L., & Husain, M. (2017b). Neurocomputational mechanisms underlying subjective valuation of effort costs. *PLoS Biology, 5*, e1002598. https://doi.org/10.1371/journal.pbio.1002598.

Cooper, J. (2007). *Cognitive dissonance: Fifty years of a classic theory*. Thousand Oaks, CA: Sage.

Croxson, P., Walton, M., O'Reilly, J., Behrens, T., & Rushworth, M. (2009). Effort based cost valuation and the human brain. *Journal of Neuroscience, 29*(14), 4531–4541. https://doi.org/10.1523/JNEUROSCI.4515-08.2009.

Dreisbach, G., & Fischer, R. (2012). Conflicts as adversive signals. *Brain and Cognition, 78*(2), 94–98.

Eisenberger, R. (1992). Learned industriousness. *Psychological Review, 99*(2), 248–267.

Eppinger, B., Hämmerer, D., & Li, S. (2011). Neuromodulation of reward-based learning and decision making in human aging. *Annals of the New York Academy of Sciences, 1235*, 1–17. https://doi.org/10.1111/j.1749-6632.2011.06230.x.

Green, L., & Myerson, J. (2004). A discounting framework for choice with delayed and probabilistic rewards. *Psychological Bulletin, 130*, 769–792.

Inzlicht, M., Shenhav, A., & Olivola, C. (2018). The effort paradox: Effort is both costly and valued. *Trends in Cognitive Science, 22*(4), 337–349. https://doi.org/10.1016/j.tics.2018.01.007.

Johnson, M., & Bickel, W. (2002). Within-subject comparison of real and hypothetical money rewards in delay dicounting. *Journal of the Experimental Analysis of Behavior, 77*, 129–146.

Kool, W., & Botvinick, M. (2014). A labor/leisure tradeoff in cognitive control. *Journal of Experiemental Psychology. General, 143*, 131–141.

Kurniawan, I., Guitart-Masip, M., Dayan, P., & Dolan, R. (2013). Effort and valuation in the brain: The effects of anticipation. *The Journal of Neuroscience, 33*(14), 6160–6169. https://doi.org/10.1523/JNEUROSCI.4777-12.2013.

Lee, D., Seo, H., & Jung, M. (2012). Neural basis of reinforcement learning and decision making. *Annual Review of Neuroscience, 35*, 287–308. https://doi.org/10.1146/annurev-neuro-062111-150512.

Levy, R., & Dubois, B. (2006). Apathy and the functional anatomy of the prefrontal cortex-basal ganglia circuits. *Cerebral Cortex, 16*(7), 916–928.

Manes, F., Sahakian, B., Clark, L., Rogers, R., Antoun, N., Aitken, M., & Robbins, T. (2002). Decision-making processes following damage to the prefrontal cortex. *Brain, 125*(Pt 3), 624–639.

Montague, P., & Berns, G. (2002). Neural economics and the biological substrates of valuation. *Neuron, 36*(2), 265–284. https://doi.org/10.1016/S0896-6273(02)00974-1.

Myerson, J., Green, L., Hanson, J., Holt, D., & Estle, S. (2003). Discounting delayed and probabilistic. *Journal of Economic Psychology, 24*, 619–635.

O'Doherty, J., Rolls, E., Bowtell, R., & McGlone, F. (2001). Representation of pleasant and aversive taste in the human brain. *Journal of Neurophysiology, 85*, 1315–1321.

Olivola, C., & Wang, S. (2016). Patience auctions: The impact of time vs. money bidding on elicited discount rates. *Experimental Economics, 19*, 864–885.

Pessiglione, M., Vinckier, F., Bouret, S., Daunizeau, J., & Le Bouc, R. (2017). Why not try harder? Computational approach to motivation deficits in neuro-psychiatric diseases. *Brain, 141*, 629–650. https://doi.org/10.1093/brain/awx278.

Peters, J., & Buchel, C. (2009). Overlapping and distinct neural systems code for subjective value during Intertemporal and risky decision making. *The Journal of Neuroscience, 29*(50), 15727–15734.

Platt, M., & Huettel, S. (2008). Risky business: the neuroeconomics of decision making under uncertainty. *Nature Neuroscience, 11*(4), 398–403. https://doi.org/10.1038/nn2062.

Prevost, C., Pessiglione, M., Metereau, C., Clery-Melin, M., & Dreher, J. (2010). Separate valuation subsystems for delay and effort decision costs. *The Journal of Neuroscience, 30*(42), 14080–14090. https://doi.org/10.1523/JNEUROSCI.2752-10.2010.

Rangel, A., Camerer, C., & Montague, P. (2008). A framework for studying the neurobiology of value-based decision making. *National Review of Neuroscience, 9*(7), 545–556. https://doi.org/10.1038/nrn2357.

Shenhav, A., Musslick, S., Lieder, F., Kool, W., Griffiths, T. L., Cohen, J. D., et al. (2017). Toward a rational and mechanistic account of mental effort. *Annual Review of Neuroscience, 40*, 99–124.

Tom, S., Fox, C., Trepel, C., & Poldrack, R. (2007). The neural basis of loss aversion in decision-making under risk. *Science, 315*, 515–518.

Walton, M., Rudebeck, P., Bannerman, D., & Rushworth, M. (2007). Calculating the cost of acting in the frotal cortex. *Annals of the New York Academy of Sciences, 1104*, 340–356. https://doi.org/10.1196/annals.1390.009.

Westbrook, A., & Braver, T. (2015). Cognitive effort: A neuroeconomic approach. *Cognitive, Affective, & Behavioral Neuroscience, 15*, 395–415.

Chapter 6
Predicting Errors and Motivation

6.1 What Is a Prediction Error and How Can It Be Used When Discussing Motivation?

Learning from this perspective, at its core, is a process by which a person can become able to use past and current events to predict what the future holds. In classical conditioning, animals learn to predict what outcomes, necessary for survival or pleasure, are contingent on which events (a buzzer sounding associated with an event or storm clouds predicting rain). The same is true for instrumental conditioning. People learn to predict the consequences of their actions, and use this knowledge to maximize the likelihood of rewards, and to minimize the occurrence of punishments. One efficient, innate way to learn to predict future reward and punishments is via error correction. The principle behind this idea is quite simple. A person makes the best prediction they can, observes actual events and if their prediction was incorrect, modify their knowledge-based stored in memory so that future predictions are more accurate.

Niv and Schoenbaum (2008) provide the following example: You are a wine connoisseur with an extensive collection of fine wines. You have your eye on a 25 -year-old wine from Bordeaux for this evening's dinner party. You predict the wine will be great as you have stored it properly. You think everything will be alright, but you never know with wine, so you are motivated to play it safe and prepare a back-up bottle just in case. When you open the wine you are thrilled to find a wonderfully complex and well-preserved example of the vintage. Though you expected this outcome, you were not sure, and were therefore actually less than 100% certain that the wine had not passed its prime. In fact, from history you knew that there was about a one-in-five chance of a bad bottle, so your prediction rate was at 80%. As a result, there is a difference between your prediction—80% chance of a good bottle of wine—and reality. You taste the bottle of wine and it is, in fact, good. You realize that your original 80% prediction might be too low. This error in prediction rate can

T. Wasserman, L. Wasserman, *Motivation, Effort, and the Neural Network Model*, Neural Network Model: Applications and Implications,
https://doi.org/10.1007/978-3-030-58724-6_6

be used to make your future prediction more accurate. Of course, not all Bordeaux are alike, so rather than update your prediction to match exactly the current situation, the prediction that all future tastings of a Bordeaux would be equally good, (100%), you might update your prediction to some other, slightly higher, probability, say 85%, rather than 80%, reflective of the higher likelihood of a good 25-year-old Bordeaux. Through this trial-and-error process of adjustment, over many bottles of wine, you will eventually learn the correct expected reward derived from different types and ages of wine. The key computational quantity that drives learning in this example is the discrepancy between predictions and outcomes. This is prediction error.

We have seen that things that have a high probabilistic value have the property of being obtainable through the effort we are willing to make. We predict the goals to be obtainable and that expectation drives selection of a particular goal to pursue. The modification of goal value through a process of prediction error analysis is one way to understand how a particular goal, objective, or value becomes motivating over time.

6.2 The Dopamine Connection

Central to any model using neuroeconomics and computational modeling to explain complex human behavior is the science that demonstrates that dopamine cells report the error in predicting expected reward delivery. Specifically, recent neuroscience discoveries show a convergence between patterns of activity in the midbrain dopamine neurons and computational model of reinforcement learning (Schultz, Dayan, & Montague, 1997). Additionally, research has shown that dopamine might also be involved in the processing of types of intrinsic motivation associated with novelty and exploration (Horvitz, 2007). This is accomplished by dopamine-based responses that are interpreted as reporting "prediction error" in general and not only "reward prediction error" in specific. Taken together, these findings support the idea that intrinsic motivation systems are represented in the brain, in part, by signals representing prediction error (Oudeyer, Kaplan, & Hafner, 2007).

Dopamine neurons come in various types, each of which are connected with distinct brain networks and have distinct roles in motivational control. Some dopamine neurons encode motivational value, supporting brain networks for seeking, evaluation, and value learning. Others encode motivational salience, supporting brain networks for orienting, cognition, and general motivation. Both types of dopamine neurons are augmented by an alerting signal involved in rapid detection of potentially important sensory cues (Bromberg-Martin, Matsumoto, & Hikosaka, 2010).

A central tenet of these models is that discrepancies between actual and expected outcomes can be used for learning. These discrepancies have been termed prediction errors and neural correlates of such prediction-error signals have been observed now in midbrain dopaminergic neurons, striatum, amygdala and even prefrontal cortex. Models incorporating prediction errors have been invoked to explain complex phenomena such as the transition from goal directed to habitual behavior, all concepts critical to the understanding of motivation and goal seeking behavior (Niv & Schoenbaum, 2008).

6.3 Reward Salience: Incentive Salience "Wanting" Versus Ordinary Wanting

Simply stated, salience is a cognitive process that confers a "desire" or "want" attribute, which includes a motivational component, to a rewarding stimulus. In our terms, it is a valuation placed upon a rewarding stimulus. Things however, are not exactly that simple. There are differences between emotionally driven (incentive salience) and more cognitive-driven types of wanting things. Cognitive wanting, in a neuroeconomic neuro-network model, depends more heavily on cortically weighted brain circuits, computationally conforms better to model-based systems, and psychologically is more tightly linked to explicit predictions of future value based on declarative remembered previous values in episodic memory (Berridge & O'Doherty, 2014). That is, if I remember liking it before, so I will like it again, to the same degree I liked it before. These cognitive desires are founded firmly on explicit representations of the predicted goodness of future outcome. That is, how much will I like it again? These predictions are usually based on declarative memories of previous pleasure of that specific outcome (Dickinson & Balleine, 2010). Dickinson and Balleine (2010) use the term utility to help explain the types of predictions that an individual will make. In these types of cognitively based desires, decision utility (in the moment decision) equals predicted utility (based upon past experience), and predicted utility is represented by remembered utility (memory of its value). In other words, a person usually is motivated by an outcome to exactly the same degree that they predict the outcome will be liked. Most predictions about future experienced utility are based on memories of how liked the outcome was in the past. We have spoken extensively about this aspect of "wanting" or motivation. This other form of wanting/motivation is called incentive salience. Its importance lies in helping us to understand how someone's current state of motivation might not be what they would predict based upon past experiences.

Incentive salience, often termed Pavlovian motivation, is a form of motivation that has several neural and psychological features that distinguish it from cognitive forms of desire. As a result of having these features, incentive salience is different, and is less rational and more emotionally driven. For incentive salience, under conditions of dopamine-related stimulation, situations exist where cue-triggered decision utility>remembered utility from the past, and similarly decision utility>predicted utility for future reward value differ (Berridge & O'Doherty, 2014). This means that it is possible to "want" what is not expected to be liked, nor remembered to be liked, as well as what is not actually liked when obtained. For example, in the past, each of us has eaten a particular pastry and enjoyed it, although we might not actually seek it out again because it is not motivating enough for us to actively seek it out. It was ok. Just nothing special. Yet, we go into the pastry shop and we see the display. The display is attractive, and the pastry looks absolutely delicious. You decide that you must have that pastry. You eat it. And you now recall that it was ok in the past, and frankly, is just ok now. Its taste did not match its cued value based upon visual presentation in the display. You now remember that in fact, you really weren't so crazy about it in the first place. In this model, incentive salience "wanting" is a pure form of decision utility, which is distinct from other forms of utility, and in some conditions can disconnect it from all the others. That is, "wanting" for an outcome is distinguishable from both experienced utility (hedonic impact or "liking" the outcome), remembered utility of how nice the outcome was in the past, and anticipated or predicted utility of how nice it will be in the future. This principle may be relevant to drug addiction as well with a person going into recovery, being released into their prior environments where the drug is readily available, and relapsing in the presence of the substance.

How Does this Happen?

Incentive salience integrates two separate input factors to generate decision utility in the moment of re-encounter with cues for a reward that could potentially be chosen based upon either a current physiological/neurobiological state or a previously learned association about the reward cue, or a Pavlovian conditioned stimulus (Berridge, 2007). These are highly automated responses that do not require cognitive reappraisal to produce their result. Something like this happens when you are walking by a restaurant, smell the food being cooked, and decide you want to eat. Issues related to this phenomenon are heavily infused in treatment for drug abuse where avoidance of triggers is an essential component of the process. When triggered by learned cues, incentive salience typically occurs as temporary peaks of motivation, relatively brief and lasting only seconds or minutes, and tied to encounters with the physical reward stimuli. Moments of vivid imagery about the reward and its cues may also serve just as well as actual physical cues to trigger incentive salience.

A particular reward cue may trigger temptation on some encounters but not on others. For example, the above mentioned food smells are more salient when you are hungry, but not so much when you have recently eaten. These alterations of the motivational power for cues help to demonstrate the difference between decision utility and predicted utility. States that alter brain dopamine reactivity can selectively alter decision utility of a reward cue (Berridge & O'Doherty, 2014). For everyone, reward cues vary in their motivational intensity across hours and days.

6.4 Dopamine in Motivation and Salience

We have seen how dopamine-based signaling in the brain is critical for a multiplicity of cognitive functions, but particular to this discussion, learning, and motivation. In the past, it was assumed that just a single dopamine signal was sufficient to support these cognitive functions, though there were competing theories as to just how this occurs. In particular there is no universally agreed upon model as to how dopamine contributes to reward-based behaviors.

Newer research has found that real-time dopamine release within the nucleus accumbens, which is a primary target of midbrain dopamine neurons, significantly varies between what have been termed core and shell subregions. The shell is the outer region of the nucleus accumbens, and, unlike the core, is considered to be part of the extended amygdala, which is located at its rostral pole. In the core, dopamine operations are consistent with learning-based theories, related to reward prediction error. In the shell, dopamine operation is consistent with motivation-based theories (e.g., incentive salience). This is logical as the placement of the shell as part of the extended amygdala makes it excellent candidate for a mediator between the two network systems. These findings demonstrate that dopamine plays multiple and complementary roles based on discrete circuits that help humans optimize rewarding behaviors. It also provides a model describing how the two networks would be engaged simultaneously, with the result being goal seeking behavior (Saddoris, Cacciapaglia, Wightman, & Carelli, 2015). The model has received research support. Research has demonstrated that basolateral amygdala (BLA) input to the core and medial shell of the Nucleus Accumbens (NAc) separately mediate two distinct incentive processes controlling the performance of goal-directed and instrumental actions, respectively: (1) the sensitivity of instrumental responding to changes in the experienced value of the goal or outcome, produced by specific satiety-induced outcome devaluation, and (2) the effect of reward-related cues on action selection, observed in outcome-specific Pavlovian-instrumental transfer. These results indicate that dissociable neural circuits involving BLA inputs to the NAc core and medial shell mediate distinct components of the incentive motivational processes controlling choice and decision-making in instrumental conditioning (Shiflet & Balleine, 2010). This research clearly indicates how prediction error networks are integrally involved in the creation and maintenance of motion.

6.5 How Prediction Error Modifies Memory

In order for this model to be operationalized it would be necessary to demonstrate how prediction error modifies memory in a way that would make certain things have more salience than others. We have looked at models that speculate on a theoretical level just how this might occur. We have also looked at indications that there are two neural systems concerned with the development and expression of adaptive behaviors: a dopamine system for reinforcement learning and a second error-processing system. The reinforcement learning function ascribed to both the dopamine system and the error-processing function appear to be focused on the same issue, evaluating the saliency of ongoing events, and then using that information to facilitate the development and expression of adaptive behaviors. There is research to suggest that the anterior cingulate cortex is a main component of the error-processing system. This error-processing system operates using error-related negativity (ERN), which is elicited when a person commits an error. ERN is generated when a negative reinforcement learning signal is conveyed to the anterior cingulate cortex via the dopamine system and this signal is then used by the anterior cingulate cortex to modify performance on the task at hand (Holroyd & Cole, 2002). We have discussed this error processing as prediction error, the difference between what we thought would happen and what actually did happen. One way for this to happen is that the dopamine-based reward system sends a negative reinforcement learning signal to the frontal cortex, where it generates the ERN by disinhibiting the specific projecting dendrites. These error signals are used to train the anterior cingulate cortex, ensuring that control over the motor system will be released to a motor controller that is best suited for the task at hand when the stimulus is next encountered.

6.6 The Human Brain Is Designed to Predict

Prediction and the modulation of expectation as a result of error analysis enable people to adapt and modify task performance so that future performance is accomplished with increasing efficiency at a minimum of effort expended. There is a distributed, bilateral network of cortical and subcortical activity supporting predictive activity (Scheidt et al., 2012). Cortical regions associated with prediction include prefrontal, parietal, and hippocampal cortices all of which are regions that are also associated with distributed working memory. Here then is a critical connection between performance-based error components related to motivation and the memory function necessary to support it.

Bilateral activations in associative regions of the striatum also demonstrate temporal correlation with the magnitude of performance error (Kawato & Gomi, 1992). Performance error has been demonstrated to be a signal that drives reward-optimizing reinforcement learning and the prospective scaling of previously learned motor and cognitive programs. These performance error signals are associated with load prediction in the cerebellar cortex and red nuclei. This is consistent with the notion that these structures generate adaptive motor signals that facilitate cancellation of expected proprioceptive feedback. This cancellation of expected feedback is required in models dealing with conditional feedback adjustments to ongoing motor commands and feedback error learning.

Research has also demonstrated that predictive activity is observed in more than one of these neural systems (Kilner, 2011; Tanaka et al., 2016). This research demonstrates that motor adaptation is mediated by predictive compensations supported by multiple, distributed, cortical, and subcortical structures. As motor adaptions are critical components of most, if not all, higher order cognitive activities it is quite likely that these distributed predictive functions are found in most processes inherent in human brain activity (Koziol, Budding, & Chidekel, 2012).

Here then, is a model for a critical, neural network based, process inherent in human motivation. Motivation is based upon probabilistic reward valuations. These valuations are developed, maintained by several processes, one of which is error predication and analysis. Error prediction and analysis allows for revaluing goals and objectives and it is valuation that drives saliency and ultimately goal selection for action. As we have seen, there are also other processes involved but error predication and modification is a core part of all of them.

References

Berridge, K. (2007). The debate over dopamine's role in reward: The case for incentive salience. *Psychopharmacology, 191*, 391–343. https://doi.org/10.1007/s00213-006-0578-x.

Berridge, K., & O'Doherty, J. (2014). From experienced utility to decision utility. In P. Glimcher & E. Fehr (Eds.), *Neuroeconomics* (2nd ed., pp. 335–351). Cambridge: Academic Press.

Bromberg-Martin, E., Matsumoto, M., & Hikosaka, O. (2010). Dopamine in motivational control: Rewarding, aversive, and alerting. *Neuron, 68*(5), 815–834. https://doi.org/10.1016/j.neuron.2010.11.022.

Dickinson, A., & Balleine, B. (2010). Hedonics: The cognitive motivational interface. In M. Kringelbach & K. Berridge (Eds.), *Pleasures of the brain* (pp. 74–84). Oxford: Oxford University Press.

Holroyd, C., & Cole, M. (2002). The neural basis of human error processing: Reinforcement learning, dopamine, and the error-related negativity. *Psychological Review, 109*(4), 679–709. https://doi.org/10.1037//0033-295X.109.4.679.

Horvitz, J. (2007). Mesolimbocortical and nigrostriatal dopamine responses to salient non-reward events. *Neuroscience, 96*(4), 1–22.

Kawato, M., & Gomi, H. (1992). A computational model of four regions of the cerebellum based on feedback-error learning. *Biological Cybernetics, 68*, 95–103.

Kilner, J. (2011). More than one pathway to action understanding. *Trends in Cogntive Neurosciences, 15*(8), 352–357. https://doi.org/10.1016/j.tics.2011.06.005.

Koziol, L., Budding, D., & Chidekel, D. (2012). From movement to thought: Executive function, embodied cognition, and the cerebellum. *Cerebellum, 11*(2), 505–525. https://doi.org/10.1007/s12311-011-0321-y.

Niv, Y., & Schoenbaum, G. (2008). Dialogues on prediction errors. *Trends in Cognitive Neuroscience, 12*(7), 265–272. https://doi.org/10.1016/j.tics.2008.03.006.

Oudeyer, P., Kaplan, F., & Hafner, V. (2007). Intrinsic motivation systems for autonomous. *Transactions on Evolutionary Computation, 11*(2), 265–286. https://doi.org/10.1109/TEVC.2006.890271.

Saddoris, M., Cacciapaglia, F., Wightman, R., & Carelli, R. (2015). Differential dopamine release dynamics in the nucleus accumbens core and shell reveal complementary signals for error prediction and incentive motivation. *The Journal of Neuroscience, 35*(33), 11572–11582. https://doi.org/10.1523/JNEUROSCI.2344-15.2015.

Scheidt, R., Zimbelman, L., Salowitz, N., Suminsky, A. J., Mosier, K. M., et al. (2012). Remembering forward: Neural correlates of memory and prediction in human motor adaptation. *NeuroImage, 59*(1), 582–600. https://doi.org/10.1016/j.neuroimage.2011.07.072.

Schultz, W., Dayan, P., & Montague, P. (1997). A neural substrate of prediction and reward. *Science, 275*, 1593–1599.

Shiflet, M., & Balleine, B. (2010). At the limbic-motor interface: Disconnection of basolateral amygdala from nucleus accumbens core and shell reveals dissociable components of incentive motivationThe European journal of neuroscience. *The European Journal of Neuroscince, 32*(10), 1735–1743. https://doi.org/10.1111/j.1460-9568.2010.07439.x.

Tanaka, S., Doya, K., Okada, G., Ueda, K., Okamoto, Y., & Yamawaki, S. (2016). Prediction of immediate and future rewards differentially recruits Cortico-basal ganglia loops. In S. Ikeda, H. Kato, F. Ohtake, & Y. Tsutsui (Eds.), *Behavioral economics of preferences, choices, and happiness* (pp. 593–616). Tokyo: Springer.

Chapter 7
Motivation Potential Is Not Motivation in Action

We have spoken about the idea that motivation represents a sort of potential to act and that the actual behavior that is motivated acts and functions, neural network wise, from its potential. Potential motivation is defined as the maximum effort an individual would be willing to exert to satisfy a motive. It is distinguished from motivation intensity, which refers to the amount of effort people actually expend (Brehm & Self, 1989). Appreciating this distinction between potential motivation and motivation intensity has been demonstrated to considerably improve the prediction of effort-related outcomes (Wright, 2008).

Take for instance the following example. It is common in consumer research to tell a subject that they have a hypothetical amount of money. Let's say that the task at hand in this study is to apportion the money between three charities each serving a particularly needy group. Descriptions of the groups are provided and then the subjects are asked to write down which charity gets how much money. They may, of course keep some for themselves. Now compare that to a situation where the subjects were actually given money and provided with descriptions of the charities. The money they gave would, of course, go to the charity. They would also have the option to keep some or all of it for themselves. Do you think the resultant distributions would be the same between the two conditions? How many variables can you think of that would influence a person's decision to part with actual money?

This is an example of a distinction that is crucial to understanding the allocation of valued resources and the relative ability to valuations to actually drive behavior. This distinction is between what individuals think that they might be willing to do to achieve a purpose and what individuals actually do to achieve that same purpose. Although action can match willingness, it often does not. We see the distinction somewhat differently. Potential, in our and others view, represents the stored, perhaps automated valuations that have been determined by inborn temperament, history, and experience. This is motivation. Behavioral action is what occurs after the motivation has determined which behavioral action to gate.

T. Wasserman, L. Wasserman, *Motivation, Effort, and the Neural Network Model*, Neural Network Model: Applications and Implications,
https://doi.org/10.1007/978-3-030-58724-6_7

7.1 The Interaction of Motivation and Effort

Brehm's model has some clear assumptions regarding the relationship of perceived required effort and motivation. The model posits that the immediate function of effort is to sustain behavior and that effort expenditure is controlled by the principle of conservation. Specifically, the more difficult the behavior required to obtain the objective, the more effort is required to sustain it. This means that effort should correspond to difficulty as long as there is a likelihood of success and effort demands do not exceed the upper limit of what people are willing to do (so long as they do not exceed potential motivation). If success seems impossible, effort should be low because its expenditure will be seen as deriving no benefit. By the same analysis, if effort demands are judged to exceed potential motivation, effort should be low because its expenditure will be seen as yielding a return of insufficient value. If the perceived required effort is too much, the individual will not try in the first place.

7.2 Initiating Motivation Potential

It would be logical at this point to ask what initiates motivation potential. What in the networked human brain moves the person from not moving toward any goal to active movement toward a specific goal? What overcomes inertia?

There are as yet no clear models that detail how this is done but we do have some clear indices about how this might occur. We know that learning how to obtain rewards requires learning about their contexts and likely causes and that long-term memory mechanisms balance the potential determinants of reward outcomes with the computational burden of an overinclusive memory. From this we can assume that here would be a way to enhance memory for salient events that occur during reward anticipation. This is because all such events are potential triggers/determinants of reward in the future (Murty & Adcock, 2014). They found that reward motivation enhances encoding of relevant events like expectancy violations. These violations occur when the expected does not happen. Fronto-cerebellar circuits are important in predicting the occurrence and timing of behaviorally relevant events and in detecting violations of predictions (expectancy violations) (Durston et al., 2007).

Specifically, motivation amplified hippocampal activation to and declarative memory for expectancy violations. This was accomplished by connectivity of the ventral tegmental area (VTA) with medial prefrontal, ventrolateral prefrontal, and visual cortices. This network preceded and predicted this increase in hippocampal sensitivity. The findings identified a discrete mechanism whereby reward motivation can enhance hippocampus-dependent memory. This network subserves anticipatory VTA-cortical–hippocampal interactions. They concluded that during reward motivation, VTA modulation induces distributed neural changes that elevate and intensify hippocampal signals and records of expectancy violations to improve predictions. It is these predictions, modified on the bases of reward experience, now stored in long-term memory that potentially represents motivation potential.

7.3 Allocation and Expenditure of Resources

Based upon what we have discussed and the empirical evidence we have reviewed thus far, it seems appropriate to utilize the ideas related to transaction cost economics to understand the allocation of resources in the human decision-making process. In economics and related disciplines, a transaction cost is a cost incurred in making an economic exchange. The same idea holds true when these ideas are utilized to model the actions of the human brain. The costs associated when decision-making processes include those involved in the expenditure of capital. In this case capital means thing like effort, attention, concentration and persistence.

By allocation of resources we mean attention, cognitive processing and behavioral action capacity that any particular person has at their disposal. A key component of the motivational decision-making process is the amount of risk (of success or failure or both) inherent in any available potential choice. Risk is just one of a number of considerations inherent in any choice. As part of the decision-making process, other variable are considered in tandem with the risk assessment. These variables include the amount of time I will have to wait to produce the outcome, the amount of effort I will have to expend, how strongly I want the outcome to occur, whether or not I need others to help me obtain the outcome and many other considerations. All these factors influence the formation of optimal allocation strategies, either by their individual or interacting effects (Jin & Zhang, 2011).

This allocation process has two overall components. The first is the easier to understand and conceptualize. This is the conscious allocation of resources on the decision factors that occur as a part of working memory. This group of factors is constrained by the limitations of human working memory, which are considerable. The second set of factors is brought into play below the threshold of human awareness. They are often referred to in the literature as unconscious factors but we have described them as previously learned, highly automated assessments. As we have seen, task-relevant cognitive or affective thought processes can occur either when the task is the focus of one's conscious attention, indicating conscious thoughts, or when one's conscious attention is directed elsewhere, standing for unconscious thought (Dijksterhuis, 2004).

Part of these automated processes includes the emotional (affective) states that have been encoded with the automated assessments of the values of previously encountered goals, objectives and values. There is research support of this hypothesis. Vroom's theory of motivation is a neuropsychological model that details processes associated with the construct. Vrooms model, called expectancy theory proposes that an individual will behave or act in a certain way because they are motivated to select a specific behavior over others due to what they expect the result of that selected behavior will be (Vroom, Porter, & Lawler, 2005). posits that people's decisions are determined by their affective reactions to certain outcomes (valences), beliefs about the relationship between actions and outcomes (expectancies), and perceptions of the association between primary and secondary outcomes (instrumentalities). This models shares many of the same characteristics with the probabilistic valuation model outlined in this book. The probabilistic model extends this work by providing a mechanism hat details how the brain actually processes the information.

One of the early major criticisms of this type of theory is that the computations it requires are unrealistically time consuming and often exceed working memory capacity. We have discussed these limitations earlier. An understanding of automaticity helps explain how the need for this type of calculation can be overcome. If an individual has extensive experience with a problem situation, he or she can process decisions about that situation using neural networks that operate implicitly (through automaticity) so that cognitive resources are not exhausted by simple computations; instead, the computations are performed implicitly by neural networks (Lord, Hanges, & Godfrey, 2003).

It is hypothesized that these affective thought processes act "as the on/off switch to motivation, which is the process by which goal-directed behavior is initiated and sustained." This affective laden motivational processing has been demonstrated to determine how learners perceive a cognitive learning task in terms of the amount of cognitive resource needed to deal with it (Schnotz & Kürschner, 2007) and goal approach behavior (Kuldas, Hashim, Hismail, Samsudin, & Abu Bakar, 2014).

7.4 The Relationship of Motivation to Emotion

We have reviewed the development of motivation earlier. It behooves us to relook at this area through the perspective of motivation potential, how it develops and how it might relate to motivated behavior. Are these points on a continuum, or are they two interrelated but distinct processes.

It is a long held view in network modeling that expressed emotions are founded/based on motivational circuits in the brain that developed early in evolutionary history to ensure the survival of individuals and their offspring. These are basic survival network circuits that react to appetitive and aversive environment (Lang & Bradley, 2010). There are psychobiological consequences of this sort of neural firing. One consequence is that they engage sensory systems that increase attention and facilitate perceptual processing of the person. This is the first step in the conversion from potential to behavioral goal seeking. Secondly, these networks are interfaced with motor networks that initiate reflex responses that mobilize the organism and prompt motor action.

Research has identified the key neural structures in this survival network. They include the bilateral amygdalae, which constitute two small, almond shaped bundles of nuclei in the temporal lobe. Each amygdala receives input from cortex and thalamus (sensory) and hippocampus (memory), subsequently engaging through the central nucleus and extended amygdala (basal nucleus of the stria terminalis) a range of other brain centers that modulate sensory processing (vigilance), increase related information processing, and activate autonomic and somatic structures that mediate defensive or appetitive actions (Davis & Lang, 2003).

This survival circuit is conceptualized as organized into two discrete motivational systems, one is defensive and is associated with unpleasant affect. The other appetitive (goal directed), associated with pleasant affect. These two motivational systems, aversive and attractive, are activated by a different unconditioned stimuli, each associated with perceptual-motor patterns and learning. Affective, goal seeking valence is determined by the more dominant appetitive system which results in positive affect. The defense system is the source of negative affect. In this system affective arousal reflects the "intensity" of motivational mobilization, determined originally by degree of survival need. The defense system is ultimately a fight or flight circuit, but in response to danger cues it also mediates behavioral "freezing" (hiding), increased vigilance, and counter-threat displays in animal subjects. The appetitive system is activated variously in alimentation, sex, and nurturance of progeny. However, as will be seen, although some reactions are uniquely appetitive or defensive, many physiological and behavioral patterns are similar in both contexts of arousal and are mediated by the same neural structures (Lang & Bradley, 2010).

This research implies that the neural network basis for motivation potential is built upon a framework of primitive flight or fight responses, established early and built upon through experience. It also implies that the basis of the advanced human construct of motivation is the primary emotional network of the human brain interacting with behavioral action networks to produce what we call motivation. This implies two interrelated but distinct processes. We should also be aware that there is research that views the primary behavioral survival reactions as the basis of all higher order cognition (Koziol, Budding, & Chidekel, 2012). That would make all motivation-related cognitions and behavior the progeny of these primary human survival mechanisms.

7.5 Value Adders and Costs

The interesting part of the Brehm's model for our discussion of motivation potential, is that it provides a way to talk about value adders and cost factors. Let's go back to our example. Let's look at what might happen if you have real money to dispense as opposed to being in a situation where you only hypothetically could dispense money. There are a number of factors that might come into play. For example, suppose a percentage of the population of subjects were poor or unemployed. They were worried about income and the ability to feed their families. Their assessment of their own need would be a powerful incentive to keep some of the money and to dispense the money differently than it would otherwise be if they did not "need" the money. Perhaps one of the subjects did not really need the money but decided that they would like a nice steak dinner that evening. The point here is that we have examples of the fact that valuation of the target goal is not the only factor to consider when discussing motivation. There are internal, intrinsic factors to consider when calculating final valuations.

Potential motivation generally excludes some situational variables as well. I can discount them easily if I want to. Motivated behavior requires much more careful consideration of the factors because I am expending actual resources. For example, if a goal can be achieved easily, then little effort should be exerted regardless of the level of willingness or potential motivation. This is a critical point to remember. We will usually, only expend the effort necessary to obtain the outcome we want. We rarely expend effort cavalierly. The difficulty of obtaining the same goal can vary considerably. Let's suppose as a child, I lived in Vale, Colorado and I love to ski. I ski every chance I get. Then I graduate high school and go the University of Hawaii. I now have to expend considerably more effort, and money, to go skiing. It is highly likely that my frequency of skiing would be much less than if I had attended the University of Colorado.

As the difficulty of goal attainment increases, so should effort, up to one of two difficulty points. The first is where success seems to be impossible (increased cost). The second is where success seems to call for more effort than would be warranted (increased risk). At and beyond these difficulty points, effort expended is likely to be low.

There is research that demonstrates this interplay of cost factors in terms of probability of success and magnitude of reward. This research demonstrates that when facing a trade-off between obtaining a higher probability of an outcome versus a higher absolute magnitude (payoff) each of which fluctuates over time, people showed a strong preference for higher probabilities of success (less likelihood of failure) over higher magnitudes (Young, Webb, Rung, & McCoy, 2014).

As we have seen, all of these factors, and many others, can be quantified and placed within a valuation model. When we speak about motivation in a neural network model, we are talking about the result of these decisional processes in relation to the determination of value of a particular goal. What we should always keep in mind is that these probabilistic value determinations are also relative to the company they keep in terms of available options for the decider to choose from.

We suppose it would be ok to have two different types of motivation. It seems more logical to understand the actual action one takes as a result of being motivated as a different construct.

References

Brehm, J., & Self, E. (1989). The intensity of motivation. In M. Rozenweig & L. Porter (Eds.), *Annual review of psychology* (pp. 109–131). Palo Alto, CA: Annual Reviews, Inc.

Davis, M., & Lang, P. E. (2003). Emotion. In M. Gallagher, & R. Nelson (Eds.), *Handbook of psychology* (Vol. 3: Biological psychology, pp. 405–439). New York: Wiley.

Dijksterhuis, A. (2004). Think different: The merits of unconscious thought in preference development. *Journal of Personality and Social Psychology, 87*, 586–598. https://doi.org/10.1037/0022-3514.87.5.586.

Durston, S., Davidson, M., Mulder, M., Spicer, J., Galvan, A., Tottenham, N., et al. (2007). Neural and behavioral correlates of expectancy violations in attention-deficit hyperactivity disorder. *Journal of Child Psychology and Psychology, 48*(9), 881–889.

Jin, X.-H., & Zhang, G. (2011). Modelling optimal risk allocation in PPP projects using artificial neural networks. *International Journal of Project Management, 29*(5), 501–603. https://doi.org/10.1016/j.ijproman.2010.07.011.

Koziol, L., Budding, D., & Chidekel, D. (2012). From movement to thought: Executive function, embodied cognition, and the cerebellum. *Cerebellum, 11*(2), 505–525. https://doi.org/10.1007/s12311-011-0321-y.

Kuldas, S., Hashim, S., Hismail, H., Samsudin, M., & Abu Bakar, Z. (2014). The unconscious allocation of cognitive resources to task-relevant and task-irrelevant thoughts. *Australian Journal of Educational & Developmental Psychology, 14*, 1–16.

Lang, P., & Bradley, M. (2010). Emotion and the motivational brain. *Biological Psychology, 84*(3), 437–450. https://doi.org/10.1016/j.biopsycho.2009.10.007.

Lord, R., Hanges, P., & Godfrey, E. (2003). Integrating neural networks into decision-making and motivational theory: Rethinking VIE theory. *Canadian Psychology, 44*(1), 21–38. https://doi.org/10.1037/h0088064.

Murty, V., & Adcock, R. (2014). Enriched encoding: Reward motivation organizes cortical networks for hippocampal detection of unexpected events. *Cerebral Cortex, 24*(8), 2160–2168. https://doi.org/10.1093/cercor/bht063.

Schnotz, W., & Kürschner, C. (2007). A reconsideration of cognitive load theory. *Educational Psychological Review, 19*, 469–508. https://doi.org/10.1007/s10648-007-9053-4.

Vroom, V., Porter, L., & Lawler, E. (2005). Expectancy theories. In J. Miner (Ed.), *Organizational behavior: Essential theories of motivation and leadership* (Vol. 1: Theories of motivation, pp. 94–113). Armonk, NY: M.E. Sharpe.

Wright, R. (2008). Refining the prediction of effort: Brehm's distinction between potential motivation and motivation intensity. *Social and Personality Psychology Compass, 2*(2), 682–701. https://doi.org/10.1111/j.1751-9004.2008.00093.

Young, M., Webb, T., Rung, J., & McCoy, A. (2014). Outcome probability versus magnitude: When waiting benefits one at the cost of the other. *PLoS One, 9*, e98996. https://doi.org/10.1371/journal.pone.0098996.

Chapter 8
Motivation: State, Trait, or Both

The question of whether the construct of motivation represents a state or a trait has significant implications for the practice of psychology. When we talk about people in general, we talk about people who appear motivated, or people who do not appear motivated. Clearly, understanding motivation as stable and consistent property of a person's behavior is an important feature in psychology. Considering motivation as a trait would allow us to measure it and perhaps make predictions about a person's future behavior. We talk about it as a trait; it is something that characterizes the behavior of a person, and something that often speaks to the character of a person.

At least sometimes we do. We all also recognize that people can be motivated by rewards, goals, and values. Child psychologists spend a good deal of time coming up with behavioral reinforcement plans to help motivate children to do their chores, listen to their parents, or finish their homework. The power of reinforcements, which are external to the person and perceived as rewarding, to motivate a person's behavior is undeniable. The ability of people to motivate themselves in situationally specific circumstances is well understood.

So which is it, or can it be both? Perhaps it is neither, or perhaps it is several different things that are best understood separately. This is a book about neural network modeling and their implications for motivation, so we will look at these questions from that perspective.

8.1 State Versus Trait

As with many things in psychology, obtaining universally agreed upon definitions of major constructs is a difficult thing to do. In general, the term state implies a temporary way of being (i.e., thinking, feeling, behaving, and relating) while a trait

T. Wasserman, L. Wasserman, *Motivation, Effort, and the Neural Network Model*, Neural Network Model: Applications and Implications,
https://doi.org/10.1007/978-3-030-58724-6_8

tends to be a more consistent, predictable, stable, enduring, and possibly automated characteristic or pattern of behavior. As an example, even a person with a well-established character trait of calmness and composure can, under the right circumstances, act agitated and angry because of being in a temporary state that is quite uncharacteristic of his or her regular style (Lazarus, 2018). These constructs are often confused, or never really specified. So if you say someone you know is nasty, are you describing the fact that they were nasty at a party or event that you heard about, or are they always nasty and have never been nice to anyone? We often ascribe personality traits to people, but do we mean that those people are always like that, or do we acknowledge that sometimes they can act differently? It may be better to describe trait as a general tendency, with exceptions. It is just not clear.

These issues have significant clinical implications. For example, when we describe a client as having trait anxiety we are implying that they are generally anxious. In contrast, state anxiety exists in a transitory emotional condition that varies in intensity and fluctuates over time. The very term "emotional state" suggests a static, unitary condition rather than a flow of continuously changing component states that constitute emotion episodes or emotional traits (Sander, Grandjean, & Scherer, 2005). On the other hand, trait anxiety refers to a stable susceptibility or a proneness to experience state anxiety frequently. One is a tendency, the other an actual physical and emotional status (Spielberger, 1972). Presaging a later discussion, one can think about a trait as a general predisposition (potential) to behave in a specific manner or demonstrate a specific behavior. State is actually experiencing or engaging in the behavior.

8.2 Motivation Is a State

Traditional conceptions of motivation describe it in a way that make it appear to somewhat goal specific and the result of some specific process. The following definitions of motivation were summarized from a variety of psychology textbooks and reflect a general consensus that motivation is an internal state or condition (Huitt, 2011). It is sometimes described as a need, desire, or want whose primary purpose is to activate or energize behavior and give it direction. Motivation was further defined as directing the arousal, direction, and persistence of behavior. These are very state-like properties in that they appear to arise in relation to some goal or situation. These definitions do not suggest a permanent condition of motivation: that a person is always motivated no matter what the circumstance. Increasingly, models are now beginning to acknowledge that the factors that energize behavior are likely different from the factors that provide for its persistence. This is a position taken in this book.

State-like conceptions are very consistent with the idea of extrinsic motivation. Extrinsic motivation refers to behavior that is driven by external rewards such as money, fame, job titles, praise, and social recognition. Extrinsic motivation emanates from stimuli outside the individual and is closely associated with operant behavioral modification approaches.

8.3 Motivation Is a State. The Role of the Basal Ganglia (BG)

In a probabilistic valuation model, this position is rather straightforward to support. As we have seen in neural network models that utilize valuation, the cerebral cortex represents the meaningfulness of multiple competing actions in separate, parallel processed, "channels." The function of the BG is to inhibit all of these channels utilizing tonically active GABAergic neurons in various BG output structures. The role of the striatum is then to disinhibit one of these channels by releasing tonic inhibition and selectively boosting activation of the most salient channel (Frank, 2011). This most salient channel is selected by means of probabilistic valuation. The probabilistic analysis would represent the motivational power of each of the available choices. The decision to pursue one option would lead to motivated approach behavior.

The BG does not select the actions themselves, but it does facilitate their execution of approach behaviors (or avoidance behaviors as we will see later) via the "direct pathway" from striatum to BG output structures. There is a secondary pathway which traverses the pallidum and subthalamic nucleus before reaching BG output structures. This pathway serves as a control process to support "capacity scaling" to ensure that no matter how many channels are active in the cortex, only one will be gated (Gurney, Prescott, & Redgrave, 2011). What gets gated is what the person is motivated to do.

In this model motivation is clearly a state because the selection process is always ongoing and always open to change. It always reflects the options available, and always represents the power and value of the eternally provided stimuli. Without internally mediated variables, the organism is always reactive, rather than internally directed.

8.4 Motivation Is a Trait

There are models of motivation that support the notion that motivation represents a trait, or a more consistent enduring state of being. (Maslow, 1943). These models suggest that motivation represents more of a personality trait, such as the need for self-actualization, which would impact much of what a person did. From a neural network perspective, for motivation to be a trait, there has to be a mechanism that allows for internally mediated consistency. This mechanism has to allow for internal "drivers" that exist in the absence of external prompts and cues. This has been described as intrinsic motivation and there is a significant literature that characterizes it (Cameron & Pierce, 2002; Rawsthorne & Elliot, 1999). Intrinsic motivation refers to engagement in behavior that is inherently satisfying or enjoyable. It is noninstrumental in nature, that is, intrinsically motivated action is not contingent upon any outcome separable from the behavior itself. Usually that means that the means and end are one and the same (Legault, 2016). There are behavioral manifestations of intrinsic motivation everywhere. People who pursue their art for its own sake, or mystics, people for whom the tenets of religion determine their moral and behavior compasses, are but a few examples. For our valuation model to work, it has to be able to explain this phenomena.

8.5 Internalized Motivation as a Trait

Self-determination Theory (SDT) (Ryan & Deci, 2000) provides a model regarding the formation and operation of intrinsic motivation. The SDT model describes how certain motivational processes become internalized to a person. Specifically, it describes the internalization characteristics of different forms of intrinsic motivation. In this model the quality of motivation is determined by the type of internalization that has taken place. There are several distinct types of internalization. Internalization can be of an intrinsic nature, because the person develops an interest for doing the activity itself and consequently finds it enjoyable. This would be an activity previously accomplished and which yielded a benefit to the person (e.g., I washed my car and it looked good). Internalization could also be of an identified nature. This form of internalization occurs when the person's regulation is transformed into a value for the outcome of the activity (e.g., I value having a clean car because of what it says about me). Internalization can also be of an "introjected" nature. This occurs when the person's regulation is internalized in its original external form (I liked cleaning my car when I was younger because that's how I earned my allowance).

The process of internalization of self-determined motivation can be understood in a probabilistic valuation model by understanding the process of automaticity. We have spoken about automaticity elsewhere (Wasserman & Wasserman, 2017). Basically, the goal of automaticity for human functioning is to conserve energy, allowing the energy to be used for addressing the novel. Humans operate using automaticity for many things. It represents the processing of information without the benefit/cost of higher order cognitive control. In this case automaticity would occur when a valuation occurred so many times, and the resulting value was so significant, that the activity, goal or value was always selected. It would then be "internalized" and operate based on internally mediated cognitions alone. Outside reinforcement would no longer be necessary. We will mention more about this process when we discuss the idea of motivation as potential. There are other ways that this internalization may come about which we will discuss below.

8.6 Motivation Does Not Always Need Goals So Maybe It's a Trait After All

Research has clearly indicated that people differ in their baseline levels of approach motivation. Relatedly, evidence suggests that approach states are not always triggered by goals; they can occur due to internal psychophysiological processes. That is, approach motivation may arise within the organism, motivating it to seek out stimuli to approach (Harmon-Jones, Harmon-Jones, & Price, 2013).

In addition, considerable research has indicated that scores on self-report measures of trait motivation of approach behavior relate to resting, baseline measures of asymmetric frontal cortical activity (Harmon-Jones, Gable, & Peterson, 2010). These results suggest the possibility of motivational temperaments influencing baseline measures in the absence of goals. A preexisting temperament, rather than goals, may motivate one to seek out a stimulus at which to be mad, or lust after.

How might these goals, objectives, or predispositions be internalized?

8.7 Motivation as State and Trait

So it seems, the construct of motivation is really a rich and complex subject. This is because it has multiple core aspects, and multiple core aspects to which the various action-selection systems are differentially sensitive. There appear to be two related but distinct main forms: goal-directed and automatic (habitual) control and both are fundamental to the study of decision making and action selection as regards motivation. The goal-directed function of motivation allows us to outline precisely outcome-specific "directing" effects. These are different from outcome-independent "energizing" effects that characterize automated responding (Niv, Joel, & Dyan, 2006).

By definition, goal-directed behavior is performed to obtain a desired goal. Although all instrumental behavior is instrumental in achieving its contingent goals, it is not, by dint of its automatic properties, necessarily specifically goal directed in its expression. Behavior is goal directed if it is both sensitive to the contingency between action and outcome, and that outcome is desired. Based on this second portion of the definition, motivation can be thought of as distinguishing between two systems of action selection. This is because if an instrumental outcome is no longer a specific valued goal, it is by definition not goal directed. It has been amply demonstrated that, after a sufficient number of trainings, the goal-directed instrumentality would fade. Extensive training can render an instrumental action independent of the value of its consequent outcome (Dickinson, 1985). This distinction between two types of behavior is also paralleled by a distinction between two different neural pathways to action selection. As we have seen, habitual behavior is thought to be dependent on the dorsolateral striatum and its dopaminergic afferents, whereas goal-directed behavior is controlled more by circuitry involving frontal cortical areas and the dorsomedial striatum. These two pathways have been suggested as subserving two action controllers with different computational characteristics, which operate in parallel during action selection. There appear to be at least two types of related, yet discrete motivational processes and perhaps there are more.

8.8 Motivation as a Continuum

Self-determination theory (Ryan & Deci, 2000) posits that there are different types of motivation, such that people vary not only in level of motivation, but also in the source or quality of that motivation. SDT highlights the fact that people operate based on internal factors such as values and ethics which do not have external valuations that produce motivated behavior. At the same time, SDT postulates a continuum of autonomy to order those types of motivation (Howard, Gagné, & Bureau, 2017). This would suggest that there was a wide range of motivational readiness dependent upon temperamental characteristics and life experience. This continuum model has a challenge. Other research (Chemolli & Gagné, 2014) suggests that motivation is best considered a multidimensional process that cannot, when considering trait-like characteristics, be represented by one valuation. This argument pushes for an analysis of motivation dependent on the context the value of the particular goal, and the history of success among other factors.

8.9 Motivation as a Partial Function of the Willingness to Accept Risk

We have spoken about the value of life course modeling in understanding how motivational traits might be developed. This model suggests that people would be born with a predisposition to behave in a motivated fashion (Reiss, 2004) that is then reinforced over time. There is research to suggest that this is possible. One way to understand what this predisposition might consist of is to look at the idea of people being born more or less comfortable with accepting risk (Demaree, DeDonno, Burns, Feldman, & Everhart, 2009). There is some research that indicates that humans and animals show variations in their ability to accept or reject risk (Grable & Joo, 2004). This might form the basis of a trait-like attitude that might develop over time. Of course, people might shift their preferences and related actions depending on the state, current needs ("state-dependent" risk attitude) or probabilistic valuations available at the time (Fujimoto & Minamimoto, 2019).

8.10 Motivation as Temperament

Research on temperament has coalesced around the idea there is a short list of core temperament dimensions. These dimensions include positive emotionality/ approach, fear, irritability/ frustration, attentional persistence, and activity level (Rothbart & Jones, 1998). If our life course/developmental model is correct, we should be able to look at these core characteristics and see how they might be built upon to produce the complex motivational behaviors that characterize human functioning.

It is well known that temperament systems follow a developmental course (Meyer, Hajcak, & Klein, 2018; Rothbart & Bates, 1998). The reactive tendencies of children to experience and express negative and positive emotions, and their responsivity to events in the environment can be observed very early in life. It is also accurate to state that these basic tendencies and the ability to regulate them and self-regulatory executive attention develops relatively late and continues to develop throughout the early school years. Because executive attention is involved in the regulation of emotions, some school children will be lacking in controls of emotion and action that other children can demonstrate with ease. As a result of attention, focus and task persistence being closely related that same developmental trajectory can be conceptualized for these skills as related to motivation.

Related research demonstrates that anxiety begins early in the course of development, and often results in chronic impairment in a variety of behavioral routines. Infants who react negatively to novel stimuli tend to become behaviorally inhibited toddlers (Fox, Snidman, Haas, Degnan, & Kagan, 2015). While the tendency toward anxiety remains relatively stable across development, its expression seems to reflect significant developmental transitions. Anxiety-related fearfulness in early childhood becomes increasingly associated with inhibition in the presence of others as children age and social interactions become more relevant (Jones, Cheek, & Briggs, 2013). As children develop we have seen how this core anxiety tends to transition from fear of external threat to self-conscious shyness and worry about behavioral competence and social evaluation (Wasserman & Wasserman, 2019). This transition between fear of concrete, external stimuli to more abstract, anticipatory, or imaginary stimuli that occurs from infancy to childhood has been proposed to be linked to changing developmental tasks and expectations.

Taken together this research point to the fact that basic goal-directed approach behaviors can be impacted by inborn temperamental characteristics that are modified by experience and circumstance. We reference elsewhere in this volume that the ability to accept and tolerate risk appears to be an essential feature of motivation. Research demonstrates that the relationship between temperamental fear- and error-related neural activity changes across development from early to middle childhood within the same individuals. Children high in temperamental fear were characterized by decreased error-related brain activity when they were approximately 6 years old (Meyer et al., 2018). Here again, the connection between early inborn predispositions and behavior related to motivation can clearly be drawn. This points to the possibility that motivation potential may represent inborn and consistent trait-like tendencies, but that motivation, when related to behavioral action, demonstrates clear state-like properties.

8.11 Motivation as the Potential to Act

Perhaps then we should be more precise about the term motivation. After all, as we have seen, motivation is not synonymous with behavior; motivation impels the organism to behave, but other considerations (e.g., motivations) may prevent the behavior from occurring (Harmon-Jones et al., 2013). We propose that motivation represents a state of readiness, or a potential, to expend effort in pursuit of either a goal, or in response to a highly automated and practiced routine, which in the past was itself goal directed.

Motivation, when operating as a trait, represents a state of readiness characterized as the highly automated and practiced approach behaviors, associated with a class of environmental stimuli. On the other hand, motivation, when operating as a state, is goal directed, that is, it is actively pursuing a particular outcome. In other words, a person is either acting in a motivated fashion, or else has the potential to demonstrate those actions if the circumstances are right. As we have seen, these represent two distinct neural networks and may be best thought of as separate processes.

References

Cameron, J., & Pierce, W. (2002). *Rewards and intrinsic motivation: Resolving the controversy*. Santa Barbara, CA: Bergin & Garvey.

Chemolli, E., & Gagné, M. (2014). Evidence against the continuum structure underlying motivation. *Psychological Assessment, 26*(2), 575–585. https://doi.org/10.1037/a0036212.

Demaree, H., DeDonno, M., Burns, K., Feldman, P., & Everhart, D. (2009). Trait dominance predicts risk-taking. *Personality and Individual Differences, 47*(5), 419–422. https://doi.org/10.1016/j.paid.2009.04.013.

Dickinson, A. (1985). Actions and habits: The development of behavioral autonomy. *Philosophical Transactions of the Royal Society B, London British Biological Science, 308*, 67–78.

Fox, N., Snidman, N., Haas, S., Degnan, K., & Kagan, J. (2015). The relations between reactivity at 4 months and behavioral inhibition in the second year: Replication across three independent samples. *Infancy, 20*(1), 98–114.

Frank, M. (2011). Computational models of motivated action selection in corticostriatal circuits. *Current Opinion in Neurobiology, 21*, 382–386. https://doi.org/10.1016/j.conb.2011.02.013.

Fujimoto, A., & Minamimoto, T. (2019). Trait and state-dependent risk attitude of monkeys measured in a single-option response task. *Frontiers in Neuroscience, 13*, 816. https://doi.org/10.3389/fnins.2019.00816.

Grable, J., & Joo, S. (2004). Environmental and biophysical factors associated with financial risk tolerance. *Journal of Financial Counseling and Planning, 15*(1). Retrieved from https://papers.ssrn.com/sol3/papers.cfm?abstract_id=2260471.

Gurney, K., Prescott, T., & Redgrave, P. (2011). A computational model ofaction selection in the basal ganglia. I. A new functional anatomy. *Biological Cybernetics, 84*, 401–410.

Harmon-Jones, E., Gable, P., & Peterson, C. (2010). The role of asymmetric frontal cortical activity in emotion-related phenomena: A review and update. *Biological Psychology, 84*, 451–462.

Harmon-Jones, E., Harmon-Jones, C., & Price, T. (2013). What is approach motivation? *Emotion Review, 5*(3), 291–295. https://doi.org/10.1177/1754073913477509.

Howard, J., Gagné, M., & Bureau, J. (2017). Testing a continuum structure of self-determined motivation: A meta-analysis. *Psychological Bulletin, 143*(12), 1346–1377. https://doi.org/10.1037/bul0000125. Retrieved from espase.curtin.edu: https://espace.curtin.edu.au/bitstream/handle/20.500.11937/69700/268067.pdf?sequence=2.

Huitt, W. (2011). *Motivation to learn: An overview*. Valdosta, GA: Valdosta State University. Educational Psychology Interactive. Retrieved from http://www.edpsycinteractive.org/topics/motivation/motivate.html.

Jones, W., Cheek, J., & Briggs, S. (2013). *Shyness: Perspectives on research and treatment*. New York: Springer.

Lazarus, C. (2018). What narcissists really think when they say… *Psychology Today*. https://www.psychologytoday.com/us/blog/think-well/201803/what-narcissists-really-think-when-they-say.

Legault, L. (2016). Intrinsic and extrinsic motivation. In V. Zeigler-Hill & T. Shackelford (Eds.), *Encyclopedia of personality and individual differences* (pp. 1–4). New York: Springer. https://doi.org/10.1007/978-3-319-28099-8_1139-1.

Maslow, A. (1943). A theory of human motivation. *Psychological Review., 50*(4), 370–396.

Meyer, A., Hajcak, G., & Klein, D. (2018). Early temperamental fearfulness and the developmental trajectory of error-related brain activity. *Developmental Psychobiology, 60*(2), 224–231.

Niv, Y., Joel, D., & Dyan, P. (2006). A normative perspective on motivation. *Trends in Cognitive Sciences, 10*(8), 1–7. https://doi.org/10.1016/j.tics.2006.06.010.

Rawsthorne, L., & Elliot, A. (1999). Achievement goals and intrinsic motivation: A meta-analytic review. *Personality and Social Psychology Review, 3*(4), 326–244.

Reiss, S. (2004). Multifaceted nature of intrinsic motivation: The theory of 16 basic desires. *Review of General Psychology, 8*(3), 179–193. https://doi.org/10.1037/1089-2680.8.3.179.

Rothbart, M., & Bates, J. (1998). Temperament. In W. Damon, & N. Eisenberg (Eds.), *Handbook of child psychology* (Vol. 3. Social, emotional, pp. 105–176). New York: Wiley.

Rothbart, M., & Jones, L. (1998). Temperament, self-regulation, and education. *School Psychology Review, 27*(4), 479–491.

Ryan, R. M., & Deci, E. L. (2000). Self-determination theory and the facilitation of intrinsic motivation, social development, and well-being. *American Psychologist, 55*, 68–78.

Sander, D., Grandjean, D., & Scherer, K. (2005). A systems approach to appraisal mechanisms in emotion. *Neural Networks, 18*, 317–352. https://doi.org/10.1016/j.neunet.2005.03.00.

Spielberger, C. (1972). *Conceptual and methodological issues in anxiety*. New York: Academic.

Wasserman, T., & Wasserman, L. (2017). *Neurocognitive learning therapy: Theory and practice*. New York: Springer.

Wasserman, T., & Wasserman, L. (2019). *Therapy and the neural network model*. New York: Springer.

Chapter 9
Motivation, Effort, and Malingering in Assessment: Similarities and Differences

There is little argument with the idea that adequate motivation is critical to learning, test taking, vocational performance, and many daily life activities (Kim, Park, Cozart, & Lee, 2015). Other activities include for example, academic achievement. As many a clinician can attest, it is quite clear that motivated students do not always actually engage in learning (Keller, 2008). This is because motivation to learn is reflective of the intention to learn or to engage in a behavior. It is only a *desire* to be involved in activities for learning and performance (Kim & Bennekin, 2013). For example, in our experience in our clinical practice with children and teens, at the beginning of the academic year, it is quite common to have the students profess their intention to do their work and study hard. They mean it. However, once the year is underway, these statements reflecting motivation are not accompanied by behaviors demonstrating action. What makes people actually learn is their mindful and purposeful engagement in those learning activities. This is because "engagement leads to outcomes such as achievement" and "motivation underpins engagement" (Martin, 2012, p. 305). One way to look at these ideas is that motivation represents intentionality, while engagement represents directed behavioral action or effort.

Motivation, effort, engagement, and by extension malingering, are terms that are often used associatively in psychology in general, and neuropsychology in particular. Remembering that these are not binary terms, rather falling along a spectrum, they are but a few of the large number of terms that have been used to describe effort, or the reason for effort, related to the performance on neuropsychological or psychological tests. Other terms have included non-optimal effort, suboptimal effort, incomplete effort, poor effort, biased responding, and negative response bias. When the effort is made in order to malinger, faking, feigning, simulating, dissimulating, magnifying, amplifying, and exaggerating are some of the terms used. Most psychologists recognize that nearly all of the above terms have been used to describe both test performance and symptom endorsement (Iverson, 2006).

T. Wasserman, L. Wasserman, *Motivation, Effort, and the Neural Network Model*, Neural Network Model: Applications and Implications,
https://doi.org/10.1007/978-3-030-58724-6_9

In addition, consideration must be given to the instances wherein underperformance or suboptimal performance may occur without the person having the specific intent to malinger or deceive. When you add in the fact that we often assess individuals with clinical conditions such as depression, which impacts effort, the business and assumptions behind effort assessment become quite complex indeed. That is, the testing may be sensitive, but not specific.

Neuropsychologists as a matter of course, estimate the extent to which a person appears to be putting forth his or her best effort during testing and then, based upon these estimates, make further inferences regarding underlying motivation to perform. A crucial component of psychological evaluations is then assessment of the effort put forth by the examinee. This assessment of effort may be even more critical in the realms of neuropsychology and forensic psychology.

Effort is not a binary phenomenon. It falls on a continuum from very poor to outstanding (Iverson, 2006). The expenditure of effort is taken to represent the degree of motivation that the examinee brings to the assessment procedure. Statements regarding effort and motivation usually are included in the reports in an attempt to state that the results of a particular evaluation accurately reflect the ability of the individual. Often these effort analyses are based on the subjective appraisal of the evaluating psychologist. Most of us have come across terms utilized in testing reports that imply that the examinee "gave his best effort" as noted by compliance and affective states. There is also the question, at the other end of the spectrum, of when a person underperforms deliberately, such as in forensic, medical, or insurance cases.

Although we might like to believe that all examinees put forth their best effort, this is not always the case. This scenario highlights a longstanding lack of conceptual clarity regarding the similarities and differences between exaggeration and poor effort when used by clinicians as descriptors in reports and research. They are clearly not the same behavioral constructs. For example, clinicians will frequently refer to poor performance on an effort test as exaggeration, describing the result of the effort rather than the effort itself. The term exaggeration is less confusing when it is used to describe symptom reporting during interview, symptom endorsement on psychological tests or behavioral observations (e.g., facial expressions, or verbal complaints of pain or fatigue). Poor effort is most often used when referencing actual behavior during testing. This simply means the person underperformed, or did not perform to their maximum, during testing. Again sensitive, but not necessarily specific. A clinician might believe or infer that this underperformance represents an exaggeration of a particular set of problems, but it is important to understand that this inference already represents a secondary clinical inference. The primary clinical inference is poor effort that is specifically directed toward a desired deceptive result. Neither of these inferences may be correct. The individual could have been tired, or bored, and wished to go home. Again, a phenomenon not unheard of in the clinical practices which includes evaluating young children.

More recently, there have been attempts to operationalize effort assessment in the form of effort probes that occur over the course of an evaluation (Heilbronner, Sweet, Morgan, Larrabee, & Mills, 2009). Effort assessment is an integral part of the effort to assess how accurate a presentation of symptomology is on the various psychological tests that comprise any battery. This phenomenon is called symptom validity assessment, utilizing symptom validity tests (SVT) and it is an important aspect of any situation where the results of the evaluations are used to qualify an individual for accommodations, school placement, or financial reward. There now exist recommendations from professional neuropsychological organizations which endorse the use of external SVT measures (Bush et al., 2005). There is as yet no absolute agreement about which ones should be used for which situation, the timing of when SVT measures should be administered in the context of other tests, how many and what guidelines should be used for interpretation. These are but a few of the serious issues involved in a discussion of SVTs and related effort (Bigler, 2014). We will assess the phenomena of symptom validity testing assessment in greater detail later.

Looked at from this perspective, neuropsychology concerns itself more with engagement and attempts to assess the level of engagement by assessing the strength of intent as reflected by motivation. Perhaps therefore, we should take a brief detour and look at what we mean when we talk about the construct of engagement.

9.1 What Is Engagement?

As we have found with many psychological constructs there is neither a simple nor agreed upon definition of engagement. It appears that engagement is a multicomponent construct, comprised of subsets of task-specific behaviors and associated indices. Engagement can be considered as what is demonstrated as cognitive and affective participation in learning activities (Kim & Bennekin, 2013). Encompassed in this definition are both cognitive engagement, defined as using shallow and deep cognitive strategies, and emotional engagement, defined as the experience of boredom, anxiety, enjoyment, and anger, for example.

There are other definitions of engagement. Fredricks, Blumenfeld, and Paris (2004) hypothesize behavioral, cognitive, and emotional engagement. Behavioral engagement describes involvement in learning tasks and environments such as time-on-task and attendance. Cognitive engagement is characterized as psychological investment in the process of learning such as the use of learning strategies. Emotional engagement describes affective reactions to learning tasks and environments such as emotions.

9.2 Terminology

Despite some overlap with the idea of emotion, neuropsychology frequently uses a number of terms, somewhat interchangeably, to describe an individual's engagement with the neuropsychology testing process. As Heilbronner et al. (2009) have noted "the neuropsychological assessment of effort, response bias, and malingering has occurred during the last 20 years. During this time various descriptors and terms have been applied to convey salient relevant concepts, sometimes in a manner that is helpful, and other times less so". While they do not mention motivation, it is often implied in the discussion of these issues. These terms are as follows:

Malingering

Malingering is the purposeful fabrication of symptoms of a mental or physical disorder. Malingering is often a consideration when doing assessment for psychological/neuropsychological status usually related to a variety of reasons such as financial gain; avoiding school, work, or military service; obtaining drugs, or as a mitigating factor for sentencing in criminal cases. When considered within the framework of a psychological or neuropsychological evaluation, a person who is malingering typically exaggerates subjective behavioral and or emotional symptomology. The person may exaggerate symptoms of depression, anxiety, pain, dizziness, sleep disturbance, memory problems, poor concentration, or personality change. During neuropsychological testing, a person who is malingering deliberately underperforms (Iverson, 2006). Malingering is not considered a medical diagnosis (Garriga, 2007).

When considering neuropsychological test performance, concerns regarding effort are frequently related or confabulated with malingering (Heilbronner et al., 2009). As we have seen, these two terms are however not the same. Merely equating less than maximal effort with malingering is a gross oversimplification. For example, an examinee who is malingering may simply put forth poor effort on neuropsychological testing as a component of his or her approach to malingering. This would be the case, for example, when an individual was claiming cognitive impairment as a result of an injury. This same examinee, when malingering, may expend considerable effort to avoid detection while being examined. Other individuals may work very diligently to feign the symptomology of a particular mental illness such as depression. Malingering is therefore multi directional and complex conceptual issue. For neuropsychologists, the process of detecting malingering also involves attention to the possibility that other disorders might be at work. Malingering must be differentiated from other entities, such as factitious disorder, conversion disorder, cogniform disorder (Delis & Wetter, 2007).

Neuropsychologists are usually interested in evaluating various parameters such as intelligence, emotional status, academic and vocational ability, and on occasion, relevant physical symptoms. To give the reader an idea of how the term malingering and effort are often confounded, we can look at the literature on malingering, specifically the purposeful, exaggeration of specific symptomology. Various terms have been used by researchers and clinicians to describe the behaviors of interest in the identification of intentionally exaggerated symptoms and diminished or reduced capability (Heilbronner et al., 2009). In particular, when examining the validity of ability measurements for example, many clinical researchers have chosen a number of different words in an attempt to imply problems with effort. These terms usually relate to purposefully underperforming. These terms include insufficient effort, inadequate effort, and poor effort. There is as yet no consensus on the preferred descriptor for test-related performance effort. The purpose of the poor effort is generally agreed upon. The term is intended to convey a purposeful and substantial negative impact on test results that results in inadequate performance. From the neuropsychologist's perspective, the result of the behavior is the invalidating of the measurement of ability relating to the particular issue at hand. This impairs the neuropsychologist who seeks to utilize such results to make accurate predictions from the data that they have collected. Clearly, this is an issue of concern. In response, neuropsychologists have created tests that are designed to evaluate the level of effort that was used in a particular assessment. Measures used to identify problematic effort are often identified as effort, which are considered to be in a category of measures that evaluate validity of symptoms, known as symptom validity tests. Clearly though, these effort tests have little to do with motivation, as the person who is engaged in malingering is usually very motivated to do poorly on the tests. Tests of effort then, at first glance, would appear to be poor assessment instruments of motivation.

Response Bias

Response bias is an example of motivated behavior which can be the polar opposite of malingering. Response bias describes the tendency for some people to present a desirable/favorable image of themselves. Often termed socially desirable responding (SDR), this tendency confounds research and forensic assessment results by creating false relationships or obscuring relationships between variables. Response bias is a major area of concern in, for example, parental fitness in custody evaluations. Each parent seeks to portray themselves as the best parent for the job (van de Mortel, 2008). It is also a major concern when using most self-report questionnaires that commonly comprise many psychological assessment batteries. Self-reporting data can be affected by an external bias secondary to social desirability or approval, especially in cases where anonymity and confidentiality cannot be guaranteed at the time of data collection. The bias in this case can be referred to as social desirability bias (Althubaiti, 2016). In response, psychometricians have created social desirability (SD) scales that are used to detect, minimize, and correct for SDR in order to improve the validity of questionnaire-based research.

9.3 Effort

At first glance, the definition of effort would appear to be straightforward. It should mention something about trying hard, or working on some elevated level of performance over baseline. For example, from the online psychological dictionary, "An effort is the activation of mental or physical power to do a task" (Pam, 2013). This definition is certainty pretty direct. There are some that are a bit more fleshed out. Mental effort was first used as a concept to help determine how hard a person tries to actively process presented information. It was seen as a combination of perceived demand characteristics, perceived self-efficacy, and level/depth of information processing such that the first two influence the last, which determines the amount of invested mental effort. These demand characteristics can easily be conceptualized as factors in a probability calculation of reward value. A related term, perceived demand characteristics depend upon the degree to which a source (e.g., a stimulus, task, context) that is being attended to poses demands on one's processing, because information has to be extracted, discriminated, remembered, and elaborated upon" (Kirschner & Kirschner, 2012). In this definition, we see the beginning of understanding the idea that the construct effort is highly task specific.

Effort has to be involved in test taking, and must in some way reflect the level of cognitive and behavioral engagement in a task. As usual with psychological constructs, the devil is in the details.

9.4 The Problems with Effort on Psychological Tests

After some brief introspection, the definition of effort, as related to test, academic or vocational activities, is not easy at all. For example, conclusions drawn from psychological tests are necessarily predicated on the notion that the individual is putting forth maximum effort to perform to the best of their ability while they are taking the test. If not putting forth good effort to perform at their best level of ability, indeed their most accurate ability level, how could assessment ever hope to evaluate an individual's ability to function (Bigler, 2014)? Instructionally, we try to insure maximum effort is made when we emphasize to every examinee something to the effect they are asked, prior to administration of any standardized neuropsychological assessment, to "do their best" or to give their "best effort" whatever that is.

Problems abound. After all, how many of us are aware of just what constitutes our best effort on any task? Isn't it at least partially accurate to state that we can always do better or try harder? How many examinees have left the testing session stating that they have left "everything on the table"?

There are of course other questions. How about if a person puts forth good but not maximum effort? What about a scenario where a person puts forth enough effort to provide a satisfactory response but knows full well that they could have tried harder? Should the caveat on most psychological reports state that the individual examinee tried hard enough, but could have done better. What is the functional difference between good enough effort representing 70% of maximum and a performance at 50% maximum? What if merely adequate effort is more than enough to solve the problem? What if maximum effort is not required? For example, most psychological tests of ability start at fairly easy levels which increase in difficulty until a person ceilings out. Many of the early questions, especially in math, have answers which are highly automated. It does not take a great deal of effort or motivation for a 10 year old to answer how much is 2 + 2. It is more accurate to say that as the level of difficulty increases so does the effort required to answer correctly. It is at least hypothetically interesting to suggest that when an individual ceilings on a test, what we are assessing is the upper limits of the effort they are willing to make on a particular task. They may, in fact, have the ability to answer, just not the desire. That would certainly make writing psychological reports more interesting. The psychologist would have to say that little "Billy stopped responding accurately at the fourth grade level. While this probably represents the limit of his academic skill set, there is some possibility that Little Billy has more skills, but was unwilling to put forth the amount of effort required to demonstrate them."

9.5 Cognitive Neuroscience and Effort

When we say effort, what is it that we are trying to represent? From a basic cognitive neuroscience perspective, effort has been estimated by manipulating several stimulus and task features, most often within working memory (attention) and short-term retention paradigms (Knight, 2007). In cognitive neuroscience research paradigms, cognitive effort may be operationally defined by task complexity and experimentally manipulated as an independent variable. In cognitive neuroscience models a bottom-up vs. top-down attention network dichotomy is used to demonstrate that only bottom-up, primary sensory stimulation engages the cortex in a manner that does not require active cognitive engagement. Bottom-up processing, is also known as stimulus-driven attention or exogenous attention. Bottom-up processing is driven by the properties of the external stimuli themselves. For example, motion or a sudden loud noise can attract our attention in a preconscious, or nonvolitional way. We attend to these stimuli whether we want to or not (Theeuwes, 1991). "Bottom-up" stimuli, especially stimuli interpreted as threats, immediately engage attentional networks, without the benefit of cognitive appraisal and are, therefore, essentially "effortless." Network components of bottom-up attention include parietal and temporal cortices, as well as the cerebellar and other brainstem features.

All other types of cognitive processes appear to require effort, no matter how insignificant or transitory the task may be, because the components of the attention and memory systems must be purposefully engaged (Bigler, 2014). All other aspects of attention require cognitive effort and a central executive (Allen, Bigler, Larsen, Goodrich-Hunsaker, & Hopkins, 2007). Studies all show that effort tests used in SVT studies measures engage the expected language, memory, attentional, and executive functioning networks necessary to perform the SVT task (Bigler, 2014). Since all SVT paradigms would seemingly utilize top-down cognitive processes, none of them, no matter how easy, could be considered effortless. On a side note, but important to our ensuing discussion, is the fact that studies actually show greater and different activation of these networks when a subject is asked to malinger. This finding suggests several things, including the facts that malingering actually takes effort, and the intriguing possibility that the neurobiology of malingering may have a signature fMRI activation profile (Kireev, Korotkov, Medvedeva, & Medvedev, 2013; Sun, Lee, & Chan, 2015).

9.6 Neural Network Models of Effort

Neural network models of effort emphasize that effort relates to the difficulty of performing a particular behavior, such as the exertion of physical force or response rate required within a limited time (Aridan, Malecek, Poldrack, & Schonberg, 2018). Network models posit that effortful behavior generally imposes a cost on valuation, revealed by discounting of rewards and preferences for less effortful alternatives. The theoretical models of valuation that are used in effort modeling suggest that the integration of expected cost and benefit representations guides choice and selection behaviors (Padoa-Schioppa, 2011). There is converging evidence linking integrated value appraisals to neural activity within a network of regions that includes the ventral striatum (VS), posterior cingulate cortex, anterior insula and ventromedial prefrontal cortex (vmPFC) (Bartra, McGuire, & Kable, 2013); and demonstrate modulation of its activity by common costs such as risk (Mohr, Biele, & Heekeren, 2010) and delay (Carter, Meyer, & Heuttel, 2010).

Human neuroimaging studies expanded the relationship of VS to effort-discounted reward and the ACC to effort-based cost–benefit analyses. Related studies also implicated primary and supplementary motor areas (SMA), insula and posterior parietal cortex as sensitive to expected effort costs. In sum, effort-based valuation studies have consistently emphasized the relationship of ACC and VS to effortful behavior, but inconsistently present several possible loci for the integration of effort and value (Aridan et al., 2018).

As can now be readily understood, the concepts of malingering and effort are quite different and should probably not be used interchangeably.

9.7 The Role of Effort in Motivation

There is a body of research that indicates that reward-driven behavior is not only regulated by factors related to the quality or quantity of reinforcement, but also by the work requirements inherent in performing instrumental actions necessary to obtain the reward in question. As a result, people often make effort-related decisions involving economic choices reflective of a cost/benefit analyses (Salamone, Correa, Yang, Rotolo, & Presby, 2018). Several neural network systems, including the mesolimbic dopamine (DA) system and other brain circuits, are involved in regulating effort-related aspects of motivation. Research indicates that mesolimbic DA transmission exerts a bidirectional control over the expenditure of effort on goal-directed behavioral tasks. Effort-based choice tasks are useful for developing animal models of some of the motivational symptoms that are seen in people with various psychiatric and neurological disorders such as depression (Yang et al., 2016), schizophrenia (Gold et al., 2013), and Parkinson's disease (Chong et al., 2015).

9.8 The Relationship of Motivation and Effort

At this point it should be clear that motivation and effort are not the same concepts. It should also be clear that estimated effort plays a role in the probabilistic reward calculation that, in a network model, might be used to represent motivation. Interestingly however, the relationship does not end there. There is evidence that motivation, which includes assessments of the amount of effort required to obtain a goal, essentially influences the amount of actual effort expended in pursuit of a goal (Goodman et al., 2011). This research demonstrated that both intrinsic and extrinsic motivation influenced the amount of effort an individual exerted in trying to achieve desired performance outcomes. The amount of effort expended by an individual was a partial mediator of the relationship between intrinsic and extrinsic motivation and academic performance. Specifically, using multiple regression analyses they demonstrated that intrinsic motivation is the strongest predictor of academic performance, followed by effort. In the regression model extrinsic motivation by itself could not explain unique variance in academic performance. In simpler terms, anticipated effort expenditure contributed to how motivated an individual was, and while motivation is critical, it is not a singular, determinant of how much effort is actually expended.

This finding is interesting from a number of perspectives. Firstly, the model again demonstrates the value of understanding motivation from a probabilistic reward calculation perspective that reflects a multiple regression equation with a number of components, the estimation of effort cost being one of them. There is research that has begun to identify what some of these variables might look like (Wittington, 2015). That study, utilizing the framework of Vroom's expectancy theory, identified three components that contribute to the development of motivation relative to a specific goal. The components are valence, expectancy, and instrumentality. Valence describes the attractiveness of a reward. Expectancy is defined as the individual's belief that his/her action would yield a specific result. Instrumentality is described as the estimated probability of individual obtaining what he/she earns.

The second idea is that motivation probably represents a range of preparatory states, and not just one absolute state that an individual has or does not have. Thirdly, motivation by itself is not sufficient to compel an individual to action. In a situation where there are a number of desirable alternative goals, each with its attendant level of motivation, one goal will be selected, while others will not be. The amount of effort may be one determinant, but it also true that things like desirability might be another.

References

Allen, M., Bigler, E., Larsen, J., Goodrich-Hunsaker, N., & Hopkins, R. (2007). Functional neuroimaging evidence for high cognitive effort on the word memory test in the absence of external incentives. *Brain Injury, 21*(13–14), 1425–1428.

Althubaiti, A. (2016). Information bias in health research: Definition, pitfalls, and adjustment methods. *Journal of Multidisciplinary Healthcare, 9*, 211–217. https://doi.org/10.2147/JMDH.S104807.

Aridan, N., Malecek, N., Poldrack, R., & Schonberg, T. (2018). Neural correlates of effort-based valuation with prospective choices. *NeuroImage, 185*, 446–454. https://doi.org/10.1016/j.neuroimage.2018.10.051. Retrieved from bioRxiv.

Bartra, O., McGuire, J., & Kable, J. (2013). The valuation system: A coordinate-based metaanalysis of BOLD fMRI experiments examining neural correlates of subjective value. *Nueroimage, 76*, 412–427.

Bigler. (2014). Effort, symptom validity testing, performance validity testing and traumatic brain injury. *Brain Injury, 28*(13–14), 1623–1638.

Bush, S., Ruff, R., Troster, A., Barth, J., Koffler, S., Pliskin, N., et al. (2005). Symptom validity assessment: Practice issues and medical necessity NAN Policy & Planning Committee. *Archives of Clinical Neuropsychology, 20*, 419–426.

Carter, R., Meyer, J., & Heuttel, S. (2010). Functional neuroimaging of intertemporal choice models: A review. *Journal of Neuroscience, Psychology, and Economics, 3*(1), 27–45.

Chong, T., Bonnelle, V., Manohar, S., Veromann, K., Muhammed, K., Tofaris, G., et al. (2015). Dopamine enhances willingness to exert effort for reward in Parkinson's disease. *Cortex, 69*, 40–46.

Delis, D., & Wetter, S. (2007). Cogniform disorder and cogniform condition: Proposed diagnoses for excessive cognitive symptoms. *Archives of Clinical Neuropsychology, 22*(5), 589–604.

Fredricks, J., Blumenfeld, P., & Paris, A. (2004). School engagement: Potential of the concept, state of evidence. *Review of Educational Research, 74*, 59–109.

Garriga, M. (2007). Malingering in the clinical setting. *Psychiatric Time, 24*(3). Retrieved from https://www.psychiatrictimes.com/articles/malingering-clinical-setting.

Gold, J., Strauss, G., Waltz, J., Robinson, B., Brown, J., & Frank, M. (2013). Negative symptoms of schizophrenia are associated with abnormal effort-cost computations. *Biological Psychiatry, 74*(2), 130–136.

Goodman, S., Jaffa, T., Keresztesi, M., Mamdani, F., Mokgatle, D., Musarir, M., et al. (2011). An investigation of the relationship between students' motivation and academic performance as mediated by effort. *South Africa Journal of Psychology, 41*(3), 373–375.

Heilbronner, R., Sweet, J., Morgan, J., Larrabee, G., & Mills, S. (2009). American Academy Of Clinical Neuropsychology consensus conference statement on the neuropsychological assessment of effort, response bias, and malingering. *The Clinical Neuropsychologist, 23*(7), 1093–1129. https://doi.org/10.1080/13854040903155063.

Iverson, G. (2006). Ethical issues associated with the assessment of exaggeration, poor effort, and malingering. *Applied Neuropsychology, 13*(2), 77–90.

Keller, J. M. (2008). An integrative theory of motivation, volition, and performance. *Technology, Instruction, Cognition, and Learning, 6*, 79–104.

Kim, C., & Bennekin, K. (2013). Design and implementation of volitional control support in mathematics courses. *Educational Technology Research & Development, 61*(5), 793–817. https://doi.org/10.1007/s11423-013-9309-2.

Kim, C., Park, S. W., Cozart, J., & Lee, H. (2015). From motivation to engagement: The role of effort regulation of virtual high school students in mathematics courses. *Educational Technology & Society, 18*(4), 261–272.

Kireev, M., Korotkov, A., Medvedeva, N., & Medvedev, S. (2013). Possible role of an error detection mechanism in brain processing of deception: PET-fMRI study. *Internal Journal of Psychophysiology, 90*(3), 291–299.

Kirschner, P., & Kirschner, F. (2012). Mental effort. In *Encyclopedia of the sciences of learning*. https://doi.org/10.1007/978-1-4419-1428-6_226. Retrieved from https://link.springer.com/referenceworkentry/10.1007%2F978-1-4419-1428-6_226.

Knight, K. (2007). Neuroscience. Neural networks debunk phrenology. *Science, 316*(5831), 1578–1579.

Martin, A. J. (2012). Commentary: Motivation and engagement: Conceptual, operational, and empirical clarity. In S. ChrChristenson, A. Reschly, & C. Wylie (Eds.), *Handbook of research on student engagement* (pp. 303–311). New York: Springer.

Mohr, P., Biele, G., & Heekeren, H. (2010). Neural processing of risk. *Journal of Neuroscience, 30*(19), 6613–6619. https://doi.org/10.1523/JNEUROSCI.0003-10.2010.

Padoa-Schioppa, C. (2011). Neurobiology of economic choice: A good-based model. *Annual Review of Neuroscience, 34*, 333–359.

Pam, N. (2013). *Effort*. Psychology dictionary. Retrieved from https://psychologydictionary.org/effort/.

Salamone, J., Correa, M., Yang, J. H., Rotolo, R., & Presby, R. (2018). Dopamine, effort-based choice, and behavioral economics: Basic and translational research. *Frontiers in Behavioral Neuroscience., 12*, 52. https://doi.org/10.3389/fnbeh.2018.00052.

Sun, D., Lee, T., & Chan, C. (2015). Unfolding the spatial and temporal neural processing of lying about face familiarity. *Cereberal Cortex, 25*(4), 927–936.

Theeuwes, J. (1991). Exogenous and endogenous control of attention: The effect of visual onsets and offsets. *Perception & Psychophysics, 49*(1), 83–90.

van de Mortel, T. (2008). Faking it: social desirability response bias in self-report research. *Australian Journal of Advanced Nursing, 25*(4), 40–48.

Wittington, K. (2015). Does Motivation Predict Persistence and Academic Success? *Open Journal of Nursing, 5*, 10–16. https://doi.org/10.4236/ojn.2015.51002.

Yang, X., Huang, J., Lan, Y., Zhu, C., Liu, X., et al. (2016). Diminished caudate and superior temporal gyrus responses to effort-based decision making in patients with first-episode major depressive disorder. *Progress in Neuropsychopharmacological Biological Psychiatry, 64*, 52–59.

Chapter 10
Disorders of Motivation

It stands to reason that if we are going to conceptualize motivation as a setoff behaviors that reflect processes in the neural network of a human brain, that, as with any other cortical process, we must allow for the fact that there are times when those processes work as they should, and times when things go awry. We are going to take a look at how issues related to motivation going awry are discussed in the extant research, and how understanding the network properties and function of motivation might lead to a reassessment of the role of motivation in disorders of mental health.

10.1 A Model for a Disorder of Motivation

The DSM 5 model of psychiatric disorders relies on grouped, clusters, of behaviors that hang together and are associated with dysfunction. These clusters yield a description of an identified disorder. Nevertheless, many recognized disorders of mental health have common elements, and one of the most commonly shared elements is disordered motivation. It is therefore, somewhat surprising to note that there are very few specific disorders of motivation listed. We have argued that a neural network interpretation for disorders of mental health will probably require a reorganization and reconceptualization of the way we think about "mental illness" (Wasserman & Wasserman, 2019) and perhaps the clearest example of this point is the consideration of the role of motivation in mental illness.

Most disorders of mental health have components reflecting poor motivation. A neural network model would argue that the *core* motivational component of all of these disorders would reflect the same neural network properties. This core network would be modified (altered, added to, or subtracted from) in some way to produce the types of disruption of functioning we see on a behavioral level related to specific "disorders." This reuse of the same core system is consistent with how the human

T. Wasserman, L. Wasserman, *Motivation, Effort, and the Neural Network Model*, Neural Network Model: Applications and Implications,
https://doi.org/10.1007/978-3-030-58724-6_10

brain evolves because the brain tends not to reinvent itself, but prefers instead to add onto what it has already utilized. It therefore stands to reason that if we could identify core network components of motivation that were common to all mental health issues, we might be able to develop treatment specifically designed to treat the motivational issue at hand. Currently this is often not the case.

In the pediatric world for example, a child typically presents for treatment for a disorder such as ADHD. The ADHD is causing trouble in school either behaviorally or with the completion of school work or both. Treaters presume that if we treat the primary disorder (improve attention) the motivation to complete school work will improve as a side benefit. The presumption appears to be that the attentional issue is blocking the natural expression of motivation. The child in question has all the motivation necessary but cannot attend to the right things in order to demonstrate this motivation. This is, however, often not the case. Improving the child's ability to attend, that is, apply their working memory to a task, does not result as a one to one correlation with improved motivation for example, to do well in school. Clinicians often have to address treatment issues for children who are compliant with their medical-based interventions for ADHD, whose overall behavior has improved in the classroom, but whose initiation of movements toward tackling classroom assignments or homework assignments remains weak. Similar analogies can be made for individuals with depression, anxiety, or OCD. Treatment targets the primary disorder and the assumption is made that motivated behavior will increase as a side benefit of the primary issue being resolved.

We are at a loss to explain why motivation has been left out as a primary disorder. Perhaps it is because motivations ubiquitous presence in most disorders, or the absence of a cogent definition, did not lend itself to the factor analytic nature of the development of the current system. In any event, we believe it is time for this to change.

10.2 The Etiology of a Motivation

Arguably, the vast proportion of people are born with neural networks that have the capacity to function normally where motivation is concerned. That is, these networks are capable of identifying environmental cues and responding to them in a manner that leads to goal seeking behavior. What then goes wrong and produces disordered motivation? We can look to certain models that reflect life course modeling for a suggestion. Specifically, what we are looking for are ideas that explain how probabilistic values fall below the critical threshold that impels goals seeking behavior.

There is research that has looked at the etiology of amotivation from both self-determination theory and social-cognitive perspectives (Hardcastle et al., 2015). Collectively, both suggest that amotivation may result from low levels of self-efficacy, outcome expectancies, effort beliefs, and value beliefs. All of these variables can be viewed from a probabilistic reward perspective as serving to diminish the value of overall valuation determination for a particular outcome or set of outcomes. Low self-efficacy refers to low confidence, and feelings by the individual that the individual lacks the capacity or resources to produce the desired behavior (the likelihood of success is low). Low outcome expectancies refers to beliefs that the costs of the behavior outweigh the benefits (the cost is too high). A lack of effort consideration is concerned with the consideration of the required amount of effort or energy needed to change behavior (it's too hard), or overcome the perceived barriers and disinhibiting factors (too much work and too hard), and being willing to invest the necessary effort to achieve the desired outcome. Finally, low value beliefs refer to not attaching sufficient value to the behavior to make it worthwhile pursuing (Wigfield & Eccles, 2000). We have seen how low outcome expectancies and value beliefs serve as demotivating factors.

In addition, the dual-process theories of action posits that behavior is driven by two processes: conscious consideration of the pros and cons, or expectancies of the value of engaging in the behavior relative to potential costs of doing so, and nonconscious processes that are spontaneous, impulsive, and occur with little deliberative thought (Hagger, Rebar, Lipp, & Chatzisarantis, 2015). We have proposed that many of these nonconscious processes should be considered from the perspective of highly automated and practiced cue-driven behavior.

10.3 Diminished Motivation and Cerebro-Cortical Damage

Disorders with associated diminished motivation have not entirely been neglected, and are in fact, receiving greater recent attention. Historically, independently demarcated disorders of diminished motivation are often noted in individuals with traumatic brain injury, and as secondary to specific disease processes. The major syndromes of diminished motivation in this regard, that have been identified are apathy, abulia, and akinetic mutism. When it comes to brain injury, depending on their etiology, disorders of diminished motivation may be a primary clinical disturbance, a symptom of another disorder, or a coexisting second disorder (Marin & Wilkosz, 2005). A good example of the issues in this section is found in Parkinson's disease. Parkinson's is caused by reduced levels of dopamine, with noted impact to motivation, affective states, cognitive states, known as non-motor areas, as well as to the more obvious motor issues. Parkinson's is may be a perfect example of wherein clinicians attempt to discriminate apathy from depression as exemplified by the administration of The Apathy Evaluation Scale (1996) and the Beck Depression Inventory (Visser, Leentjens, Marinus, Stiggelbout, & van Hilten, 2006) to assist with a discriminative diagnosis in many research studies.

Most literature on brain injury conceptualizes disorders of motivation on a continuum of motivational loss, with apathy at the minor pole of severity and akinetic mutism at the major pole of severity. These disorders result from dysfunction of the neural machinery that mediates motivation (American Congress of Rehabilitation Medicine, 1995). This is somewhat, but importantly different than depression. In depression, one feels sad. An absence of motivation or apathy however, reflects an absence of emotion. In other words, these disorders occur when the neural network that subserves motivation is actually broken. They were described as follows:

Apathy: Apathy is a state of reduced motivation in a state of normal consciousness, attention, cognitive capacity, and mood. Patients with apathy are generally able to initiate and sustain behavior, describe their plans, goals, and interests, and react emotionally to significant events and experiences. However, these features are less extensive, less common, less intense, and shorter in duration than they are in individuals who are not apathetic. In specific, apathy differs from normality quantitatively rather than qualitatively (Marin & Wilkosz, 2005).

Abulia: Abulia originally referenced a disorder of will, which characterized people with symptoms less severe than, but qualitatively identical to, akinetic mutism. These symptoms included poverty of behavior and speech output, lack of initiative, loss of emotional responses, psychomotor slowing, and prolonged speech latency (Berrios & Gili, 1995).

Akinetic Mutism: Akinetic mutism is essentially characterized by a total absence of spontaneous behavior and speech occurring in the presence of preserved visual tracking (Mega & Cohenour, 1997).

10.4 The Effect of Disrupted Motivation on Daily Functioning

Motivation can also be disrupted when the brain has not been identifiably damaged. Historically, motivation without obvious, associated brain injury is a psychological construct defined by goal-directed behavior. In a diminished capacity, poor motivational levels impact daily functioning across ages, environments, and affectual states. As it currently stands, the assessment of motivation in clinical settings is by extrapolation. Assessment requires examining goal-related aspects of overt behavior, thought content, and emotion. In this regard, disorders of diminished motivation are identified by the simultaneous diminution in each of these three aspects of behavior:

Diminished overt behavior may range from a subtle reduction in social or occupational functioning, to symptoms of diminished overt behavior including diminished productivity, diminished effort, and diminished initiative.

Mildly diminished goal-related thought content was identified by decreased interests, plans, or goals for the future. When severe, these symptoms escalated to a virtual absence of goal-related thought content. The latter would characterize abulia and akinetic mutism.

Diminished emotional responses to goal-related events indicate emotionally indifferent, shallow, or restricted responses to important life events. Clinically, this usually means flattened, labile, or shallow affect and emotional indifference.

When viewed as a collection, these three aspects of motivational deficiency could be seen as prongs of a spectrum of disorders ranging from mild to severe. These disorders could be diagnosable, and treatable in their own right.

As we have highlighted multiple times, the impact of disordered motivation may be more focused and specific. For example, we have suggested elsewhere that certain forms of attentional deficit disorder are better understood in terms of motivated arousal (Wasserman & Wasserman, 2015). The current authors have made a point (2015) in highlighting how misdirected attention is the result of disrupted motivation rather than disrupted attention circuitry. That is, the authors maintain that the children are paying attention, simply not to that which we are asking them to direct their attention, as they find other activities, environmental or internal, of greater reward value, which motivates them to direct their attention in those stimuli instead.

This leads to a fundamental and as yet unanswered question. Contrary to the idea of disrupted attention impacting motivation, can it be disrupted motivation impacting the direction of attention? A similar argument can be made regarding OCD wherein for example, cleaning behavior takes on greater probabilistic reward value, perpetuates the behavior and becomes the motivational guide. In both of these examples, it is important to note that the hyper focused motivation in the specific examples outlined, results in a relatively absent, or diminished level of motivation for other pursuits. As an aside, we are not suggesting that all cases of ADHD are due to disordered motivation. We have seen cases in clinical practice where attention is truly disrupted. We are saying that some are due to disordered motivation and the meshing these two groups in research means that potentially meaningful findings are obscured or missed entirely.

10.5 Disrupted Motivation in Various Psychiatric Conditions and Associated Neural Network Components

Support for a neural network interpretation for the role of motivation being disrupted in disorders of mental health come from a number of studies. For example, specific motivational and emotional regulatory functions have clearly defined neural circuitry (Best, Williams, & Coccaro, 2002). Specifically, this line of research has demonstrated that the lateral orbitofrontal (OFC) and the ventromedial PFC (including orbital) (VMPFC) regulate emotion and motivation (Price, Carmichael, & Drevets, 1996). There is research that suggests that damage to these specific circuits produces disordered motivation and emotional regulation (Arsten & Rubia, 2012) or engagements.

Relatedly, there is ample evidence of the role of prefrontal cortical (PFC) networks in the behavior and cognitive functions that are impacted in childhood neurodevelopmental disorders (Arsten & Rubia, 2012). The PFC structures "top–down" regulation of attention, inhibition/cognitive control, motivation, and emotion through networked connections with multiple posterior cortical and subcortical structures. Dorsolateral and inferior PFC regulate attention and cognitive/inhibitory control, whereas orbital and ventromedial structures regulate motivation and affect. Neuroimaging studies of children with a variety of neurodevelopmental disorders that have motivational components show altered brain structure and function in specific circuits with respect to these functions. For example, children with attention-deficit/hyperactivity disorder show specific abnormalities in the inferior PFC and its connections to striatal, cerebellar, and parietal regions. Children with conduct disorder show alterations in the paralimbic system, comprising ventromedial, lateral orbitofrontal, and superior temporal cortices together with specific underlying limbic regions which regulate motivation and emotion control. Children with major depressive disorder show alterations in ventral orbital and limbic activity, particularly in the left hemisphere, mediating emotions. Finally, children with obsessive compulsive disorder appear to have a dysregulation in orbito-fronto-striatal inhibitory control pathways, but also deficits in dorsolateral fronto-parietal systems of attention.

Disrupted motivation can also be found in depressive disorder (Pizzagalli, Losifescu, Hallett, Ratner, & Favab, 2008) and in aging (Eppinger, Hämmerer, & Li, 2011). Further, there is ample evidence of the disruption of motivation-driven goal seeking behavior in schizophrenia (Barch & Dowd, 2010). Messinger et al. (2011) describe two sub-domains of negative symptoms in schizophrenia: diminished expression which includes blunted affect, and motivational deficits which is a decrease in goal-directed behavior associated with a decrease in curiosity and interest. There is recent research that suggests that anhedonia is specifically associated with decreased motivation for rewards. Specifically, anhedonia is generally assumed to reflect aberrant motivation and reward responsivity (Treadway, Buckholtz, Schwartzman, Lambert, & Zald, 2009). In fact, there are motivational issues that underlie most disorders of mental health. Doesn't it stand to reason that motivation, and the specific disorders associated with it, should be identified and targeted specifically?

10.6 Athymhormia and Disorders of Motivation in Basal Ganglia Disease

The idea that disordered motivation may, in fact represent a distinct class of emotional regulatory difficulties worthy of its own diagnostic consideration is not new. Habib (2004) conceptualized human motivation as a separate function lying at the interface between emotion and action. According to this model, motivation can be ascribed to subcortical circuits that are mainly centered on a subset of the basal ganglia and on their limbic connections.

Neuroanatomical modeling of theses circuits, between the basal ganglia and frontal cortex, indicates that these cortico-subcortical connections are organized in several loops functioning in parallel. Each, hypothetically, subserves a discrete function (Alexander & Crutcher, 1990). Alexander described five parallel cortico-subcortical loops originating from, and terminating in different parts of the frontal cortex. One of these circuits, mainly originating in the anterior cingulate cortex, encompasses the ventral striatum, the ventral part of the globus pallidus and the posteromedial medial-dorsal nucleus of the thalamus, and then projects back again to the anterior cingulate. This circuit, connecting cortical and subcortical components of the limbic system, is involved in motivational and emotional control. There is considerable, converging evidence to consider the limbic (or ventral) striato-pallidum as an "interface between motivation and action" (Mogenson, Jones, & Yim, 1980). As we have discussed earlier, if motivation represents the potential for action based on historically determined and automated probabilistic reward assessments, there would need to be a system to convert these stored assessments from probability to action. The limbic striato-pallidum is the candidate site for this conversion of motivational processes into behavioral output (Apicella, Ljundberg, Scarnati, & Schultz, 1991). This idea is buttressed by the observation that the limbic striato-pallidum receives afferents from the amygdala, which is involved in emotional labeling of sensory stimuli, and from the hippocampal formation, which compares incoming information with past experience, and then projects to the rest of the basal ganglia mass, involved in initiating and organizing motor acts (Salamone, 1994).

In sum, we are left with a few questions. Is the lack of a set of specific motivational disorders a function of history? Might it be wise to consider such a set of diagnoses? Many of the children seen in treatment are referred because they are under motivated and poorly performing in school. Standard practice is to diagnose a disorder that is the presumed cause of the motivational deficiency, and treat that disorder with the expectation that motivation is improved as a result. Might we have this process backward? It is worth taking a look.

10.7 Disrupted Motivation in Mental Health

Much of this work is based on the idea that the neural networks underpinning motivated behavior would be disrupted in some manner, thereby producing the resultant motivational disruption. If we are to consider a mental health diagnosis, separate and apart from brain injury, then we must conjecture how the network system may be dysfunctional, while still remaining intact. Fortunately, there is a way to do this.

To assess the impact of motivational states on mental health diagnoses, one must identify a neural network that interconnects systems that analyze, maintain in long-term memory and retrieve the affective value of a given stimulus or contextual cue. As we have seen, this process is subserved by the amygdala-hippocampus-orbital-frontal system. This retrieval process must be interfaced with systems that control movement initiation, mental activity, and emotional expression. These operations are conducted in various parts of the basal ganglia, under the form of separate frontal-subcortical loops.

We have already identified the amygdala as a contributing structural site of association between stimulus and reward (Murray, 2007). This research demonstrates that there are two systems within the amygdala, operating in parallel, that enable reward-predicting cues to influence behavior. The first one mediates a general, arousing effect of reward, and the other links the sensory properties of reward to emotion. There are strong projections from the amygdala to the limbic striatum, and network connections between limbic and motor parts of the striatum point to the limbic striato-pallidum for the role of converting affective representations contained in the amygdala into motor routines. The limbic part of the striatum would represent the driving center of the three main discrete fronto-striatal loops operating in tandem. Each loop possesses a specific output (motor acts for the motor loop, emotional expression for the limbic loop, and spontaneous mental activity for the associative one), accounting for the three main symptoms of the athymhormic syndrome. According to this representation, damage, or less than optimal performance to the limbic loop, while leaving intact the other two loops, would result in impaired spontaneous cognitive and motor activity, giving rise to the characteristic symptoms of athymhormia: lack of spontaneous action (despite intact motor functioning) and poverty of spontaneous thinking in the presence of preserved intellectual capacities (Habib, 2004).

This systematic representation provides a plausible explanation for the type of a motivated behavior most clinicians see in their offices. What is left to work out, is how and why this particular network component would become inefficient in its task. However, what we do have is a clear, identifiable, and testable hypothesis that could serve as the underpinning for a diagnosis of a disorder of motivation. As we have written about in detail elsewhere (Wasserman & Wasserman, 2017), life course modeling provides a plausible developmental pathway that would describe the various factors that would contribute to the functional operation of a particular network component.

10.8 Self-Determination Theory

One way that we might understand how a nosology of motivational disorders might be generated is to take a second look at self-determination theory (SDT). SDT hypothesizes a continuum of motivational types ranging from most to least self-determined. The most self-determined types are intrinsically motivated, and the least self-determined types are extrinsic. There is also recognition that an individual might be amotivated (Deci & Ryan, 1985, 2000). Self-determined motivation references performing an action out of choice, rather than out of external obligation or internal pressure. Intrinsic motivation is the most self-determined form of motivation, and refers to doing an activity for the pleasure and satisfaction derived from participation. Extrinsic motivation encompasses behaviors that are linked to a separable outcome, and comprises four behavioral regulations. Integrated regulation is the most self-determined form of extrinsic motivation and includes behaviors that are consistent with a person's self and value system. Identified regulation represents actions that are performed out of choice, though they are not attractive in and of themselves (i.e., practicing scales on a piano in preparation for a concert). Introjected regulation exists when a person internalizes, but does not endorse, external forces (e.g., going to an office party to avoid being thought of as someone who didn't want to be part of the team). Finally, external regulation refers to behaviors that are regulated by external sources (i.e., a child cleaning their room in order to get their allowance).

Overall, autonomous motivation incorporates actions that are taken volitionally, and, therefore, comprises intrinsic motivation, integrated regulation, and identified regulation. In contrast, controlled motivation involves intra- or interpersonal coercion, and therefore includes introjected and external regulations. Finally, amotivation falls at the least self-determined end of the motivational continuum, and is defined as a lack of intention of act (Sheehan, Herring, & Campbell, 2018).

Clearly, the idea that an individual can be amotivated or poorly motivated in their own right is both logical and accepted. The amotivated state in particular would seem to be very impairing and could arguably be recognized as a disorder of mental health. Just as clearly, all of the other motivational states might be efficient in their operation or, as a result of life course issues, be inefficient in their own right. They do not have to be attached to another disorder to be impairing, and we do not necessarily need to understand the other disorder to understand why the person is dysfunctional.

10.9 Life Course Modeling and the Development of Motivation

In brief, life course modeling focuses on the idiosyncratic adaptive capacity of individuals to optimize development across major changes over their life course. This adaptive capacity relies on the learned ability to self-regulate motivational processes. This self-regulatory skill is developed though selecting, adapting, and pursuing developmental and personal goals that reflect responses changing life course opportunities. These motivational self-regulatory skills involve anticipating emergent opportunities for goal pursuit, activating behavioral and motivational strategies of goal engagement, disengaging from goals that have become futile and/or too costly, and replacing them with more feasible and timely goals (Heckhausen, Wrosch, & Schulz, 2010).

Life course modeling proposes four major topics to consider when looking at the developing the efficiency of the motivational network system:

(a) Adaptiveness of primary control which are processes that are conceptualized as directed at changing the world to bring the environment into line with one's wishes.
(b) Life span trajectories of primary and secondary control. Secondary control processes are defined as changing the self to bring oneself into line with environmental forces.

(c) Optimization of goal choice and accordant use of control strategies.
(d) Action phases of goal choice, goal engagement, goal disengagement, and goal reengagement.

Problems can go wrong in the development of competence in any of these areas, and when they do, dysfunctional or poorly adaptive motivational behavior can occur. Interfacing the life course model with the development of the neural network responsible for the operation of the resultant motivational processes, should allow us to develop plausible models of motivational development, and the disordered behavior that occurs when the process does not occur as expected.

10.10 Disordered Motivation and Drug Addiction, a Clue to the Basis of a Motivational Disorder

Drug addiction is often viewed as the final step in a series of transitions from initial voluntary, sporadic drug use, to regular but "controlled" use, finally terminating in compulsive, uncontrolled usage (Everitt & Robbins, 2005). There is a line of research that considers this to be result of a motivational disorder in which the desire for the drugs themselves overpowers the drive to attain most other nondrug rewards (Goldstein et al., 2007). Motivation to seek rewards is evoked by stimuli associated with reward availability (cues). Neural networks associated with the mesocorticolimbic reward system, and particularly the ventral striatum, mediate incentive salience to stimuli associated with reward availability. This is true for all reward seeking behavior including the use of drugs.

The incentive-sensitization theory of drug addiction posits that these neural circuits become, through the processes of automization, hypersensitive to drug-associated stimuli (Robinson & Berridge, 2003). This results in amplified incentive salience of drug cues compared with nondrug cues. This might lead to increased probability of drug-seeking and drug-taking behavior, and decreased probability of nondrug-related behaviors.

Additional research found that an imbalance in the incentive salience of drug-relative to nondrug-reward-predicting stimuli in dependent compared with nondependent smokers in a network that drives subsequent motivation to obtain the respective reward could represent a central mechanism of nicotine addiction. This research suggested that preventive approaches and therapeutic treatments that aim to enhance the salience of nondrug-reward-predicting stimuli in addicts could be effective in relapse prevention (Bühler et al., 2010).

We offer this example, not as an in depth analysis of drug addiction, which it clearly is not but rather, a suggestion that the root cause of the problem lies in the disruption of motivation that is not caused by cerebral insult. What's more, it suggests that the treatment be directly related to restoring the normal balance of motivation for cues unrelated to the drugs. In other words, treat the motivational issues or more specifically, treat the disordered motivation.

10.11 Summary and Directions

Collectively, neural network modeling provide clear direction regarding the conditions that lead to the development of amotivation and how they could be addressed. As we have conjectured, based on these findings, strategies aiming to reduce amotivation could include confidence-building strategies, targeting decisional balance and also those that focus on changing effort and value beliefs. These strategies should therefore be part of any clinical treatment plan where being poorly motivated is at issue.

The fact is that these types of strategies are often used in counseling approaches to changing behavior. Techniques such as motivational interviewing (Miller & Rollnick, 2013) have directly targeted motivation as part of a therapeutic change process. This line of research argues persuasively that motivational deficiencies should be targeted in their own right as clinically handicapping conditions.

The important point for this discussion is that disruption of motivation is an essential component of many disorders of mental health. Despite its ubiquitous presence, in the current nosology it hardly ever stands on its own. However, the question becomes why doesn't disordered motivation have its own set of specific mental health diagnoses? Is it possible that motivation serves as the core of many disorders of mental health and our current focus on the other disorders as having preeminence is misplaced? We think this might be the case.

References

Alexander, G., & Crutcher, M. (1990). Functional architecture of basal ganglia circuits: Neural substrates of parallel processing. *Trends in Neurological Science, 13*, 266–271.

American Congress of Rehabilitation Medicine. (1995). Recommendations for use of uniform nomenclature pertinent to patients with severe alterations in. *Archives Physical Medicine and Rehabilitation, 76*, 205–209.

Apicella, P., Ljundberg, T., Scarnati, E., & Schultz, W. (1991). Responses to reward in monkey dorsal and ventral striatum. *Experimental Brain Research, 85*, 491–500.

Arsten, S., & Rubia, K. (2012). Neurobiological circuits regulating, attention, cognitive control, motivation, and emotion: Disruptions in neurodevelopmental psychiatric disorders. *Journal of the American Academy of Child & Adolescent Psychiatry, 51*(4), 356–367. https://doi.org/10.1016/j.jaac.2012.01.008.

Barch, D., & Dowd, E. (2010). Goal representations and motivational drive in schizophrenia: The role of prefrontal–striatal interactions. *Schizophrenia Bulletin, 36*(5), 919–934. https://doi.org/10.1093/schbul/sbq068.

Berrios, G., & Gili, M. (1995). Abulia and impulsiveness revisited: a conceptual history. *Acta Psychiatrica Scandinavica, 92*, 161–167.

Best, M., Williams, J., & Coccaro, E. (2002). Evidence for a dysfunctional prefrontal circuit in patients with an impulsive aggressive disorder. *Poceedings of the National Academy of Sciences, 99*, 8448–8453.

Bühler, M., Vollstädt-Klein, S., Kobiella, A., Budde, H., Reed, L., & Braus, D. (2010). Nicotine dependence is characterized by disordered reward processing in a network driving motivation. *Biological Psychiatry, 67*, 745–752. https://doi.org/10.1016/j.biopsych.2009.10.029.

Deci, E. L., & Ryan, R. M. (1985). *Intrinsic motivation and self-determination in human behaviour*. New York: Plenum Press.

Deci, E. L., & Ryan, R. M. (2000). The "what" and "why" of goal pursuits: Human needs and the self-determination of behavior. *Psychological Inquiry, 11*, 227–268. https://doi.org/10.1207/S15327965PLI1104_01.

Eppinger, B., Hämmerer, D., & Li, S. (2011). Neuromodulation of reward-based learning and decision making in human aging. *Annals of the New York Academy of Sciences, 1235*, 1–17. https://doi.org/10.1111/j.1749-6632.2011.06230.x.

Everitt, B., & Robbins, T. (2005). Neural systems of reinforcement for drug addiction: From actions to habits to compulsion. *Nature Neuroscience, 8*, 1481–1489.

Goldstein, R., Alia-Klein, N., Tomasi, D., Zhang, L., Cottone, L., Maloney, T., et al. (2007). Is decreased prefrontal cortical sensitivity to monetary reward associated with impaired motivation and self-control in cocaine addiction. *American Journal of Psychiatry, 164*, 43–51.

Habib, M. (2004). Athymhormia and disorders of motivation in basal ganglia disease. *The Journal of Neuropsychiatry and Clinical Neurosciences, 16*, 509–524.

Hagger, M., Rebar, A. M., Lipp, O., & Chatzisarantis, N. (2015). The subjective experience of habit captured by self-report indexes may lead to inaccuracies in the measurement of habitual action. *Health Psychology Review, 9*(3), 296–302. https://doi.org/10.1080/17437199.17432014.17959728.

Hardcastle, S., Handcox, J., Hattar, A., Maxwell-Smith, C., Thøgersen-Ntoumani, C., & Haggar, M. (2015). Motivating the unmotivated: How can health behavior be changed in those unwilling to change? *Frontiers in Psychology, 6*, 835. https://doi.org/10.3389/fpsyg.2015.00835.

Heckhausen, J., Wrosch, C., & Schulz, R. (2010). A motivational theory of life-span development. *Psychological Review, 117*(1), 32. https://doi.org/10.1037/a0017668.

Marin, R., & Wilkosz, P. (2005). Disorders of diminished motivation. *The Journal of Head Trauma Rehabilitation, 20*(4), 377–388. https://doi.org/10.1097/00001199-200507000-00009.

Mega, M., & Cohenour, R. (1997). Akinetic mutism: Disconnection of frontal-subcortical circuits. *Neuropsychiatry Neuropsychology and Behavioral Neurology, 10*, 254–259.

Messinger, J. W., Trémeau, F., Antonius, D., Mendelsohn, E., Prudent, V., et al. (2011). Avolition and expressive deficits capture negative symptom phenomenology: Implications for DSM-5 and schizophrenia research. *Clinical Psychology Review, 31*, 161–168.

Miller, W., & Rollnick, S. (2013). *Motivational interviewing: Preparing people for change* (3rd ed.). New York: Guildford.

Mogenson, G., Jones, D., & Yim, C. (1980). From motivation to action functional interface between the limbic system and the motor system. *Progress in Neurobology, 14*, 69–97.

Murray, E. (2007). The amygdala, reward and emotion. *Trends in Cognitive Sciences, 11*(11), 489–497. https://doi.org/10.1016/j.tics.2007.08.013.

Pizzagalli, D., Losifescu, D., Hallett, L., Ratner, K., & Favab, M. (2008). Reduced hedonic capacity in major depressive disorder: Evidence from a probabilistic reward task. *Journal of Psychiatry Research, 43*, 76–87. https://doi.org/10.1016/j.jpsychires.2008.03.001.

Price, J., Carmichael, S., & Drevets, W. (1996). Networks related to the orbital and medial prefrontal cortex; a substrate for emotional behavior. *Progress in Brain Research, 107*, 523–536.

Robinson, T., & Berridge, K. (2003). Addiction. *Annual Review of Psychology, 54*, 25–53.

Salamone, J. (1994). The involvement of nucleus accumbens dopamine. *Brain Behavior Research, 61*, 117–133.

Sheehan, R., Herring, M., & Campbell, M. (2018). Associations between motivation and mental health in sport: A test of the hierarchical model of intrinsic and extrinsic motivation. *Frontiers in Psychology, 9*, 707. https://doi.org/10.3389/fpsyg.2018.00707.

Treadway, M., Buckholtz, J., Schwartzman, A., Lambert, W., & Zald, D. (2009). Worth the 'EEfRT'? The effort expenditure for rewards task as an objective measure of motivation and anhedonia. *PLOS One, 4*, e6598. https://doi.org/10.1371/journal.pone.0006598.

Visser, M., Leentjens, A. F., Marinus, J., Stiggelbout, A. M., & van Hilten, J. J. (2006). Reliability and validity of the Beck depression inventory in patients with Parkinson's disease. *Movement Disorders, 21*, 668–672.

Wasserman, T., & Wasserman, L. (2015). The misnomer of attention deficit hyperactivity disorder. *Applied Neuropsychology: Child, 4*, 116–122. https://doi.org/10.1080/21622965.2015.1005487.

Wasserman, T., & Wasserman, L. (2017). *Neurocognitive learning therapy: Theory and practice*. New York: Springer.

Wasserman, T., & Wasserman, L. (2019). *Therapy and the neural network model*. New York: Springer.

Wigfield, A., & Eccles, J. (2000). Expectancy-value theory of achievement motivation. *Contemporary Educational Psychology, 25*, 68–81. https://doi.org/10.1006/ceps.1999.1015.

Chapter 11
How to Motivate People

There is of course an extensive body of literature regarding people and how to motivate them. Some of this material is for academic purposes and some for commercial endeavors. There are numerous theories about motivation, and many models that are proposed about how people develop and sustain motivation. These models talk about things that motivate. They often detail both intrinsic and extrinsic factors that motivate people. For the most part, we look at intrinsically held values as somewhat immutable and resistant to change. Arguably, the process of getting a person to change these intrinsic values would be both long and arduous. This is a concept which sweeps across disciplines and industries including sociology, fund raising, marketing, and politics to name a few. On the other hand, extrinsic motivation is simpler to understand from a probabilistic valuation model: Change the perceived value of the available extrinsic options and you can change the goal seeking behavior of the individual. Behavior therapists have recognized this for a long time. As clinicians well know, child psychologists have a long history of successfully modifying behavior; by showing parents how providing powerful incentives for their children regarding a highly desired parental choice of a behavior can produce behavioral changes in the child. This leads to a number of questions including the obvious one: Is motivating people by altering extrinsic motivation the same as motivating them by altering intrinsic processes?

We have argued that intrinsic motivation represents inborn temperamental core characteristics that are developed and modified over the life course by experience of success and failure. We have pointed out that part of these automated processes include the emotional (affective) states that have been encoded with the automated assessments of the values of previously encountered goals, objectives and values. We have seen how Vrooms model, called expectancy theory proposes that an individual will behave or act in a certain way because they are motivated to select a specific behavior over others secondary to what their expectation of the result of that selected behavior (Vroom, Porter, & Lawler, 2005). This theory includes the idea that people's decisions are determined by their affective reactions to certain out-

T. Wasserman, L. Wasserman, *Motivation, Effort, and the Neural Network Model*, Neural Network Model: Applications and Implications,
https://doi.org/10.1007/978-3-030-58724-6_11

comes (valences), beliefs about the relationship between actions and outcomes (expectancies), and perceptions of the association between primary and secondary outcomes (instrumentalities).

If this model is accurate, we can the conjecture that the modification of extrinsically valued goals and intrinsically valued goals would be governed by the same processes. They would differ as to the required frequency, intensity, and duration of the intervention process. Clearly, undoing automated preset intrinsic goals and objectives would also involve undoing previously held valuations in addition to generating new valuation assessments.

11.1 Processes that Alter Valuation Determinations

Change is hard, and the concept of change is usually anxiety producing. In fact, evidence from a number of studies indicates that people are loss averse: they dislike losses much more than they enjoy equal-sized gains (Ericson & Fuster, 2011). Therefore, given a choice, people will tend to stay where they are, or hold onto their beliefs, rather than change them.

The idea that valuations are impacted by uncertainty, and change, although with some difficulty, is supported by research into the effects of drug addiction on the valuations of other potential goal selections. Selective changes in responses to uncertainty have been observed in response to intoxication and deprivation from various drugs of abuse. We have seen that uncertainty is a powerful determinant of motivated behavior. Research has demonstrated that drug users deprived of their drug of choice, displayed reduced valuation of uncertain rewards, especially when these rewards were more objectively valuable. This uncertainty aversion increased with increasing quantity of drug use. This reduction in the valuation of uncertain rewards decreases motivated behavior for most other goals and objectives other than the drug of choice (Hefner, Starr, & Curtin, 2016), the known entity. This devaluation of rewards of objective value then, is offered as part of the explanation for both continued substance use and relapses.

Similarly, research with pathological gamblers showed increased discounting of delayed rewards and a trend toward decreased discounting of probabilistic rewards. At the neural network level, gamblers exhibited increased delay discounting and decreased probability discounting neural value correlations in the reward system (Miedl, Peters, & Büchel, 2012).

So we have examples of how a pattern of naturally motivating events can be altered into a pattern where only one highly motivating event or choice dictates a person's behavior. We also have then an idea of what it might take to alter long held beliefs and values. It would take a highly rewarding, highly stimulating alternative reinforcer that is initially external in nature, but over time is internalized and automated to become a powerful intrinsic reward. This notion has significant meaning for the process of therapy. To alter behavior, similar conditions might need to be created. Clearly, this would be difficult using verbal persuasion alone. Might there be other ways to alter long held valuations?

11.2 Stress and Altered Probabilistic Valuation

There is substantive research that demonstrates that stress has an impact on probabilistic valuations. A wide range of stressful experiences can influence human decision-making in complex ways beyond the simple predictions of a fight-or-flight model. Research suggests that stress exposure influences basic neural circuits involved in reward processing and learning, while at the same time biasing decisions toward habit, and modulating our propensity to engage in risk-taking (Porcelli & Delgado, 2017).

The impact of stress is seen along three vectors that interact with each other. These factors are stress-to-task latency, stressor duration, and exposure across the lifespan. For instance, a few minutes difference in latency can be enough to influence stress effects on risk-taking, a key component of motivation. Similarly, stressors that are repeated or occur long-term become chronic, and have been associated with structural changes in decision-making. Stress effects have also been demonstrated based on the lifespan phase of the individual. Adolescents exposed to early life stress, for example, are susceptible to changes in affective/motivational circuits typically involved in decision-making (Porcelli & Delgado, 2017). In sum, stress research highlights three general trends; acute stress can impair valuation of reward information critical to decision-making, acute stress influences a shift from goal-directed to habit-based decision-making and effects of acute stress on risk-taking are mixed depending on the length of the acute stress and the value of the reward.

This line of research clearly suggests that the reduction of chronic stress is a key element in preparing a person for motivational change. It also indicates that people have a propensity to devalue goals and objectives while they are stressed and, as a result, be less likely rather than more likely to change. This also goes a long way to explain why individuals in high stakes testing situations are more likely to view the situation as beyond their control. All of this points to suggest that in high-stress situations, activities that promise mastery and an increased possibility of success would bring about the likelihood of generating more behavior that was motivated to change and accomplish the task.

11.3 Self-Efficacy and Motivational Change

There is some evidence that supports this idea. The basic model comes from Bandura (1977) and states that many types of psychological procedures alter the level and strength of a person's set of competence relative to a specific outcome. These expectations of personal efficacy determine whether approach behavior will be initiated, how much effort will be expended, and how long it will be sustained in the face of obstacles and aversive experiences. Persistence in activities that are perceived as threatening but in fact relatively safe produces, through experiences of mastery, further enhancement of self-efficacy and corresponding reductions in defensive and avoidant behavior. Probabilistic valuations will be altered in the direction of trying to obtain the goal and motivation for that goal will be accomplished. This makes observable sense. For example, think about a scenario wherein a person falls in a body of water and is struggling. Your perception or appraisal of your strengths as a swimmer will become critical in your decision-making process. Logically, the person who has practiced this life saving exercise under more controlled conditions, and repeatedly been successful, will more likely to not experience the avoidance, but rather, be more likely to engage. In Bandura's model, expectations of personal efficacy are derived from four principal sources of information: performance accomplishments, vicarious experience, verbal persuasion, and physiological states. The more dependable the experiential sources, the greater are the changes in perceived self-efficacy.

To be clear, Bandura did not talk about probabilistic valuations, we added that part of the discussion. Probabilistic network modeling explains what Bandura observed; we are extending or updating the model and making the connection. What Bandura noted on a behavioral level, is explainable and understandable on a neural network level using the neural economic conceptions we have been speaking about. To presage the discussion a bit, behavioral change is best accomplished through behavioral practice. Several studies have demonstrated the superiority of behavioral mastery as opposed to other forms of externally imposed valuation modifying methods. For example, in a study that examined the influence of different sources of efficacy information on self-efficacy strength, results indicated that a performance accomplishment led to significantly stronger efficacy than did observation of a model, which in turn was more effective in strengthening efficacy than was hearing a verbal message. Second, performance accomplishment strengthened efficacy even when it followed one or both of the other sources of efficacy information. Finally, a verbal persuasion message was most effective in strengthening efficacy when it followed a performance accomplishment (Wise & Trunnel, 2001). Let's take a look at each of these factors in turn.

11.4 Self-Efficacy Redefined

Before we look at each of the component factors that strengthen or alter self-efficacy let's look at the concept itself, and see how it relates to the neuroeconomic, probabilistic valuation model we are describing.

"Self-efficacy beliefs influence how people think, feel, motivate themselves, and act. Self-efficacy is concerned about the perception or judgment of being able to accomplish a specific goal and cannot be sensed globally. In order to gain a sense of self-efficacy, a person can complete a skill successfully, observe someone else doing a task successfully, acquire positive feedback about completing a task, or rely on physiological cues" (Zulkosky, 2009, p. 93). Self-efficacy makes a difference in how people feel, think, behave, and most importantly for us, motivate themselves. A low sense of self-efficacy is associated with stress, depression, anxiety, and helplessness. People with self-esteem become pessimistic about their accomplishments and personal development. As regards thinking, a high sense of efficacy facilitates cognitive processes and performance, including quality of decision making and academic achievement. Self-efficacy influences people's choice of activities. Self-efficacy levels can increase or diminish motivation. People with high self-efficacy approach difficult tasks as challenges and do not try to avoid them. People's self-efficacy beliefs determine their level of motivation, as reflected in how much effort they will exert in an endeavor and how long they will persevere in the face of obstacles (Bandura, 1989). In other words, people with high self-esteem relative to a specific goal or objective, behave in a motivated fashion, and people with low self-esteem do not.

A way to understand self-esteem as regards neural network modeling, is to think about the fact that people who have high self-esteem relative to a task have a higher probabilistic valuation that they will be successful in accomplishing the task. That valuation will be based on history, the desirability of the goal or object and how specifically successful the individual has been in accomplishing the task before. People with high self-esteem (high expectation of success) are motivated. People with low self-esteem are people whose expectation for success is so low that they are not impelled to action. They are not motivated. Like probabilistic valuations, self-efficacy is specific to the goal, objective, or value it is referencing. It is true that some people may believe themselves to be efficacious in many situations, and other people hardly feel efficacious at all. No one believes themselves efficacious in all situations. The same factors that go into calculating the probabilistic calculation for likelihood of success go into the creation of self-efficacy. In other words, the probabilistic valuation model explains the concept of self-efficacy pretty well.

Now that we understand that, we can look at the power of various mechanisms designed to alter self-efficacy and speculate that they would operate in a similar fashion when talking about altering probabilistic valuations.

There is some research evidence that supports this line of reasoning. This research suggests that belief in one's ability to exert control over the environment and to produce desired results is essential for an individual's well-being, and that the perception of control is not only desirable, but it is likely a psychological and biological necessity. This same research suggests that the need for control is a biological imperative for survival, and a corticostriatal network is implicated as the neural substrate of this adaptive behavior (Leotti, Iyengar, & Ochsner, 2010). The prefrontal cortex and the striatum play important roles in perceiving control. As noted elsewhere in this book, these regions form a corticostriatal network that produce the motivational states associated with control and choice. The ability to choose is considered an inborn trait for humans. How it develops depends upon experience.

More recently, the neural network components and properties of self-esteem have become elucidated. This research is based on the idea that self-esteem is shaped by the appraisals we receive from others. There is a computational model that functionalizes this relationship by capturing fluctuations in self-esteem created by prediction errors that quantify the difference between expected and received social feedback. These social prediction errors are associated with activity in ventral striatum/subgenual anterior cingulate cortex, while updates in self-esteem resulting from these errors covaried with activity in ventromedial prefrontal cortex (vmPFC). Of interest and importance, these are the same prediction error systems that operate in probabilistic valuation.

This research linked computational parameters to psychiatric symptoms and identified an "interpersonal vulnerability" dimension. Symptoms of depression, social anxiety, and trait and state anxiety showed a positive association with "interpersonal vulnerability." Once defined this vulnerability modulated the expression of prediction error responses in anterior insula and insula vmPFC connectivity during self-esteem updates (Will, Rutledge, Moutoussis, & Dolan, 2017).

Finally, there is research that looks at the effect of reward on self-efficacy that indicates that reward for self-efficacy operates in the same fashion as does reward for probabilistic valuation. Specifically, when reward is high, self-efficacy has a positive effect on performance, whereas when reward is low, it has a negative effect. This suggests that reward moderates the effect of self-efficacy on performance (Tzur, Ganzach, & Pazy, 2016).

11.5 Performance Accomplishments, Self-Esteem, and Motivation

We have already seen how actually performing an action to achieve or obtain a goal provides the best boost in future goal seeking behavior and motivation. Self-efficacy is enhanced by practicing the intended behavior or task. Experiences of success are the most effective way to develop a strong sense of self-efficacy. Seasoned firefighters must have a strong sense of self-efficacy in order to engage in a literal environmental blaze. These experiences provide evidence that a person can succeed and show the exertions that success costs. Negative experiences disrupt the feeling of self-efficacy, especially when a failure takes place before a stabile sense of self-efficacy has been developed (van de Laar & van de Bijl, 2001).

There is increasing evidence that effort by itself, and successful effort in particular, improves goal seeking behavior, and by implication, motivation for future similar situations. For example, research suggests that the amount of effort we put into accomplishing a task exerts a positive influence on subsequent reward processing and outcome evaluation. Specifically, the mere making of an effort toward a particular reward increases subjective evaluation toward subsequent similar reward (Ma, Meng, Wang, & Shen, 2014). There is also clear evidence that efforts a critical variable in cognitive choice. Neural representations of the effort utilized in performing actions, and the valuations of the outcomes they yield, form the foundation of action choice. We have seen that there are specific neural networks that exist to assess the amount of effort required to obtain a goal. Specifically, how anterior cingulate cortex and dorsal striatum (dorsal putamen) signaled the anticipation of effort independently of the prospect of winning or losing or potential valuation. We indicated that activity in ventral striatum (ventral putamen) was greater for better-than-expected outcomes compared with worse-than-expected outcomes, an effect modulated by greater exerted effort. Therefore, neural representations of anticipated actions are sensitive to the expected demands, but not to the expected value of their consequence, whereas representations of outcome value are discounted by exertion, commensurate with an integration of cost and benefit so as to approximate net value (Kurniawan, Guitart-Masip, Dayan, & Dolan, 2013). Therefore these effort networks are clearly delineated and provide a key component to the development and maintenance of motivation.

11.6 Vicarious Learning, Self-Esteem, and Motivation

Vicarious learning, involves observing other persons' experiences and learning from them. The observer's own capacities are then assessed in relation to that other persons' successes and failures. Seeing comparable others persist and succeed in a difficult task strengthens the idea that the observer can do it themselves. As a corollary, seeing others fail in spite of hard efforts can strengthen the observer's doubts about their own capabilities. Vicarious learning works best when the observer views themselves as very similar to the person they are observing. This lack of direct experience makes vicarious learning less powerful in altering behavior.

Compatibility assessments are based on two criteria: shared experiences and similar personal characteristics. Persons with a comparable lifestyle, like friends or colleagues, can serve as models, and models can show skills for the intended behavior. Models who succeed slowly, by trial and error, are better than those who succeed instantly, without problems. Some models can be counterproductive; for instance, models with many more capabilities are usually deemed too dissimilar.

Similar characteristics also have a positive influence, although these characteristics may have nothing to do with the behavior at issue. Comparability in sex, age, ethnic background, socioeconomic status, or educational level usually are seen as indicators of a person's own capacities (van de Laar & van de Bijl, 2001). All of these indicate that valuation assessments of the model are based on the models similarities with the observer. The closer the similarity, the greater value is placed on the learning experience as being instructive. This extra step of valuing the model inevitably leads to some discounting of the model because a perfect match is not possible. This inherently implies that vicarious methods have less power than direct experience.

11.7 Verbal Persuasion, Self-Esteem, and Motivation

Verbal persuasion is the most commonly used source of information for enhancing/ modifying self-efficacy. It also serves as the basis for most forms of psychotherapy. Verbal persuasion is used to tell people that they have the capability to succeed, or the ability to learn how to succeed. This is because data suggest that people will have more confidence in themselves if others have confidence in their capabilities. In therapy, it is assumed that this encouragement via verbal persuasion causes patients to make more efforts and persevere in a task until the desired behavior has been mastered. While these self-strengthening suggestions have been shown to enhance the development of skills and eventually self-efficacy, they have limited power when used in isolation. Verbal persuasion is best used in combination with other methods (Bandura, 1997).

Verbal persuasion has been found to produce other potential benefits. It may also help people to set higher goals than they would have done by themselves. It should be pointed out that the goals that are being encouraged should remain realistic and attainable. Research demonstrates that goals that are not realistic result in patients getting discouraged by disappointing results. Positive feedback can also be viewed as a kind of persuasion (Gonzales, Goeppinger, & Lorig, 1990). Positive feedback has been demonstrated to be an important reward to induce patients to show a specific behavior and keep it up. As attribution theory would suggest, it is also important, of course, to attribute success to the patient's own efforts (Graham, 1990; Heider, 1958).

The probability of success of persuasive communication in changing beliefs associated with behavior change is strongly associated with the assessed reliability of the source (Montano & Kasprzyk, 2015). The more reliable the person who is communicating the message is assessed to be, the greater the likelihood of success in changing attitudes or learning a new behavior. As we have seen, this assessment of reliability is based on three factors: expertise, credibility, and attractiveness (Klucharev, Smidts, & Fernández, 2008). These are the same factors that the probabilistic valuation model uses to establish reliability (Cusella, 1982). Patients experience more feelings of efficacy if they are convinced by a reliable person than if the person is someone they do not trust. In addition, the communicator's reliability is enhanced when they are perceived as knowledgeable on the topic (Bandura, 1997).

11.8 Self-Appraisal of Emotional and Physiological Responses, Self-Efficacy, and Motivation

The fourth source of self-efficacy is the information people obtain from self-appraisal of their physiological and emotional situation. As we have seen, people who feel stressed will judge their self-efficacy more negatively than persons who feel relaxed. Similarly, a positive mood increases self-efficacy and a negative mood decreases it (van de Laar & van de Bijl, 2001). Self-efficacy can be increased by improving the patient's physical situation, reducing stress, and decreasing negative emotions, as well as by correcting false interpretations of the patient's physical situation. The intensity of emotional and physical reactions is not as important as the way they are observed and interpreted. When persons have high self-efficacy, they see a certain tension as a stimulant to achieve, but persons who have doubts experience tension as a restraint. Finally, people have more confidence in their abilities (appraise their skills at a higher level) when they are relaxed (Maddux, 1995). We have seen how stress impacts probabilistic valuation in much the same manner (Porcelli & Delgado, 2017).

Depending on one's perspective, physical symptoms can be viewed as indicators of personal ineffectiveness, and changing these interpretations is important. Cognitive behavioral approaches to treatment base their effectiveness on their ability to have people reinterpret these symptoms in a way that leads to greater adaption (Ellis & Dryden, 1987). Of course, it should be stressed that it isn't called cognitive behavioral therapy as the person is encouraged to practice new behaviors that derive from these new beliefs. As in probabilistic valuation change, competent behavior drives self-esteem.

11.9 What Is the Relationship of Self-Esteem and Motivation?

We should point out from the beginning of this discussion, that the relationships between self-esteem, motivation, and other constructs that describe elements of goal seeking behavior have not yet been clearly elucidated in the research literature. Self-efficacy is clearly similar to both effort–performance expectancy (a form of motivation) and the performance–outcome expectancy (another form of motivation described in the literature). Both motivational constructs and self-efficacy hypothesize that successful performance depends on effort. Self-efficacy beliefs are similar to the effort performance motivation based on the perceptions of the relationship between the degree of effort put forth and the level of performance. There are also several differences between these constructs. First, compared to effort-performance, self-efficacy beliefs are based on a broader domain of perceptions such as personal ability, skills, knowledge, previous task experience, and complexity of the task to be performed, as well as on the states of psychomotor reactions. Second, self-efficacy includes the idea of generative capability (e.g., a proficient football player may believe that they would make a good football coach for children). Third, self-efficacy distinguishes between several construct and measurement dimensions (e.g., strength, magnitude, generality, composite) where the motivational constructs are more specific (Stajkovic & Luthans, 2003).

11.10 Motivation as a Continuum

We have seen how self-determination theory (Deci & Ryan, 2000) posits that there are different types of motivation, and that people vary not only in level of motivation, but also in the source or quality of that motivation. In other words, the components of motivation and their levels vary from person to person. This variation creates the likelihood that there is a continuum of motivation and related motivated behavior throughout the population. Clearly, this idea is attractive to psychologists and neuropsychologists who desire to measure motivation.

The way that children learn motivation is important to consider because understanding the process allows us to identify methods to utilize that would instill certain values and perhaps eliminate others. While the processes are considered to be inborn, as we have seen, internalization is determined by personal history (success or failure), activity characteristics, and context. These vary idiosyncratically, with the result being that the regulation of a particular behavior can be internalized in different ways, ranging from remaining completely external (therefore not internalized), to being regulated by internal pressures, to being completely self-regulated. In sum, the quality of motivation is determined by the type of internalization that has taken place (Chemolli & Gagné, 2014). Clearly then, successful mastery experiences would be key to the process of improving motivation.

We should point out that there is data to suggest that the continuum model may not be the best way to conceptualize motivation. For example, if motivational regulations were to differ in degree, instead of kind as the continuum hypothesis hypothesizes, these motivational regulations should yield a single dimension when using factor analytic techniques, at the very least when trying to obtain second-order factors. To date, the factor structure obtained from past research all indicate multidimensional solutions, where each latent factor represents one of the regulations (Mallett, Kawabata, Newcombe, Otero-Forero, & Jackson, 2007; Tremblay, Blanchard, Taylor, Pelletier, & Villeneuve, 2009).

If motivation were to differ only in degree as opposed to kind, a person could only "be" on one location on the continuum at any given time. Research fails to support this model. It demonstrates that, if we offer people several reasons for engaging in an activity that reflects the different types of motivation, people usually endorse more than one reason (Chemolli & Gagné, 2014).

All of this serves to suggest that motivation is likely not a uniform, single construct but rather a group of interrelated covarying constructs that are highly related to a specific goal, idea, or value. More recent research provides clarifying information between the continuum vs. non-continuum models. This research demonstrates clearer support for a core continuum structure of motivation, though this continuum is not completely in line with the way it is postulated in SDT. This is because criterion-related tests revealed that relying solely on a single latent motivation construct results in the loss of critical information specific to each motivation type. In other words, relying on a single construct representing quantity of self-determined motivation is insufficient to fully explain all motivational covariates pertinent to a particular situation (Howard, Gagné, Morin, & Forrest, 2016). In sum, while there is a core of motivation that is common to all motivated behavior, it seems quite likely that the elements of motivated behavior vary from target to target within the same person. For example, one may go to work because they are highly motivated to get paid, but they love going skiing, although no one is paying them to do it.

11.11 Motivation Is Best Assessed in Relation to a Specific Target or Goal

All of the above signals that motivation is best assessed in relation to a specific target goal, value, or objective. In addition, improving a person's motivation is best accomplished by generating an improved sense of mastery in relation to the specific target, goal, value or objective in question. For example, intrinsic motivation is significantly correlated with academic achievement (mastery) in students with learning difficulties (Wery & Thomson, 2013) and motivational general-mastery imagery has been shown to increase self-efficacy and related performance among athletes (Parkerson, Harris, Langdon, & Czech, 2015). Overall, research on variables related to academic success has found that motivation, self-efficacy, and value-expectancy are the most highly correlated influencing factors on student academic behavior. These variables are in turn heavily influenced by how students experience success, confidence and well-being, lecturers' motivation and enthusiasm, and how theory and practice is tied together (Nilsen, 2009).

Of course, this all has significant implications for clinical practice. For example, let's say your patient is a somewhat asocial and clumsy individual who has trouble talking to people. Typically, one possible course of action is to send that patient to one of the many social support groups for socially awkward people that are available in your community. In fact, your client goes, and practices speaking with other individuals who similarly require social skills. While this is a great first step, it may not be successful in convincing your client to go and make attempts to socialize in the community at large. Most often you hear, "Those people *have* to talk to me" as the reason why the group behavior led to conversation, but also the reason why your client continues to refuse to try outside the group setting. Motivation is somewhat specific to the target. Again, successful mastery experiences with the actual target are a key determiner of improving motivation (Poulsen, Rodger, & Ziviani, 2006). The implications here regarding self-efficacy, and by extension self-esteem, are self-evident.

While Bandura spoke about self-esteem as a driver of motivation, it is very enticing when viewing the construct through the lens of a neuroeconomic model, to view self-esteem as a proxy for talking about motivation itself. It is certainly true that the techniques for improving self-esteem are understandable in terms of probabilistic valuation modeling and have been demonstrated to actually improve motivation-like behavior. As we have seen reframing self-esteem using probabilistic valuation modeling is pretty straightforward. Doing so allows you to map self-esteem onto known properties of specific neural networks and allows for a solid biological foundation for the construct. We have spoken at length about ideas such as probabilistic reward valuation, error analysis, goals, and effort. How might these ideas be presented to the public at large?

We thought it might be interesting to look at how popular motivational speakers talk about motivation in a way that is easily understandable in terms of these same neural network concepts. We take a few of these "popular ideas" and then reinterpret them from a neural network perspective. We went to the literature and pulled out some popular and well-known quotes. The following come from Tony Robbins (2020). They are good examples of reframing, using error analysis, cost valuation, overcoming inertia, and reward networks. Of course, by virtue of the fact that someone is enrolling in one of these motivational workshops or buying the books, implies that this person is somewhat motivated to make changes. That is, perhaps motivational coaching works because of the state of the person when they engage. Nonetheless, the elements of self-efficacy, reward valuation, overcoming inertia, error analysis, and effort are all implied.

1. "If you do what you have always done, you'll get what you have always gotten." This quote hits on a number of major themes. First and foremost that people have a desire for sameness and learn to accept outcomes that may be less than optimal. Secondly, improving motivation is about making change, and that change is difficult.
2. "Every problem is a gift, without problems we would not grow." This quote encourages the listener to redefine problems as opportunities. Problems are considered to be difficult to solve and the expectation for solving them is low. Opportunities imply a higher probability of success and a higher expectation of reward. Higher reward increases probabilistic valuation.
3. "The meeting of preparation with opportunity generates the offspring we call luck." This statement supports the idea that practice increases the likelihood of a successful outcome and that successful practice increases the probability of success in the future.
4. "It is in your moments of decision that your destiny is shaped." Active decision-making is critical for the development of motivation.
5. "A real decision is measured by the fact that you've taken a new action. If there's no action, you haven't truly decided." Action is essential for the development of motivation. It is not sufficient to think about doing something or to imagine yourself doing it. You must actively move toward a goal in integrated and successful steps.
6. You see, in life, lots of people know what to do, but few people actually do what they know. Knowing is not enough! You must take action." See above. Implicit in all of this is that one should not be afraid to make errors as they are an essential part of learning. Errors are educational and necessary.
7. "The only thing that's keeping you from getting what you want is the story you keep telling yourself." This implies that if a person has a low expectation of success they will not try. Remember that is not sufficient to want a goal, you have to believe that you have the capacity and skill to obtain that goal.
8. "Success in life is the result of good judgment. Good judgment is usually the result of experience. Experience is usually the result of bad judgment." This suggests that making errors is a critical and necessary part of the development of motivation. Our judgment improves based upon what we have learned from our mistakes.

9. "People are not lazy, they simply have impotent goals. That is goals that do not inspire them." Lack of motivation is the result of goals that do not have sufficient valuation to cause the assignment of effort.
10. "If you talk about it, it's a dream, if you envision it, it's possible, but if you schedule it, it's real." See number 6. Effort is an essential component of motivation.
11. "The more rejection you get, the better you are, the more you've learned, the closer you are to your outcome… If you can handle rejection, you'll learn to get everything you want". See 6, 8, and 12.
12. "Take the opportunity to learn from your mistakes: find the cause of your problem and eliminate it. Don't try to be perfect; just be an excellent example of being human." Again, analysis of errors and the modification of behavior, based on error analyses, to more closely approximate success is an essential component in the development of motivation. Again of course, we have self-efficacy and reframing as well.

Once you understand neural network modeling, much of what is written about motivation can be understood from that perspective.

References

Bandura, A. (1977). Self-efficacy: Toward a unifying theory of behavioral change. *Psychological Review, 84*(2), 191–215.

Bandura, A. (1989). Human agency in social cognitive theory. *American Psychologist, 44*, 1175–1184.

Bandura, A. (1997). *Self-efficacy, the exercise of control*. New York: W.H. Freeman.

Chemolli, E., & Gagné, M. (2014). Evidence against the continuum structure underlying motivation measures derived from self-determination theory. *Psychological Assessment, 26*, 575–585. https://doi.org/10.1037/a0036212.

Cusella, L. (1982). The effects of source expertise and feedback valence on intrinsic motivation. *Human Communication Research, 9*(1), 17–32. https://doi.org/10.1111/j.1468-2958.1982.tb00680.x.

Deci, E. L., & Ryan, R. M. (2000). The "what" and "why" of goal pursuits: Human needs and the self-determination of behavior. *Psychological Inquiry, 11*, 227–268. https://doi.org/10.1207/S15327965PLI1104_01.

Ellis, A., & Dryden, W. (1987). *The practice of rational emotive therapy*. New York: Springer.

Ericson, K., & Fuster, A. (2011). Expectations as endowments: Evidence on reference-dependent preferences. In R. Ahluwalia, T. Chartrand, & R. Ratner (Eds.), *Advances in consumer research* (Vol. 39, pp. 142–143). Duluth, MN: Association for Consumer Research.

Gonzales, V., Goeppinger, J., & Lorig, K. (1990). Four psychosocial theories and their application to patient education and clinical practice. *Arthritis & Rheumotolgy, 3*(3), 132–143. https://doi.org/10.1002/art.1790030305.

Graham, F. (1990). *Attribution theory: Applications to achievement, mental health, and interpersonal conflict*. New York: Lawrence Erlbaum. isbn:978-0-8058-0531-4.

Hefner, K., Starr, M., & Curtin, J. (2016). Altered subjective reward valuation among drug-deprived heavy marijuana users: Aversion to uncertainty. *Journal of Abnormal Psychology, 125*(1), 138–150. https://doi.org/10.1037/abn0000106.

Heider, F. (1958). *The psychology of interpersonal relations*. New York: Wiley. isbn:978-0-8985-9282-5.

Howard, J., Gagné, M., Morin, A., & Forrest, J. (2016). Using bifactor exploratory structural equation modeling to test for a continuum structure of motivation. *Journal of Management, 44*, 2638–2664. https://doi.org/10.1177/0149206316645653.

Klucharev, V., Smidts, A., & Fernández, G. (2008). Brain mechanisms of persuasion: How 'expert power' modulates memory and attitudes. *Social Cognitive and Affective Neuroscience, 3*(4), 353–366. https://doi.org/10.1093/scan/nsn022.

Kurniawan, I., Guitart-Masip, M., Dayan, P., & Dolan, R. (2013). Effort and valuation in the brain: The effects of anticipation and execution. *The Journal of Neuroscience, 33*(14), 6160–6169.

Leotti, L., Iyengar, S., & Ochsner, K. (2010). Born to choose: The origins and value of the need for control. *Trends in Cognitive Neuroscience, 14*(10), 457–463. https://doi.org/10.1016/j.tics.2010.08.001.

Ma, Q., Meng, L., Wang, L., & Shen, Q. (2014). I endeavor to make it: Effort increases valuation of subsequent monetary reward. *Behavioural Brain Research, 261*, 1–7.

Maddux, J. (1995). *Self-efficacy, adaptation, and adjustment: Theory, research, and application*. New York: Springer.

Mallett, C., Kawabata, M., Newcombe, P., Otero-Forero, A., & Jackson, S. (2007). Sport motivation scale-6 (SMS-6): A revised six-factor sport motivation scale. *Psychology of Sport and Exercise, 8*, 600–614. https://doi.org/10.1016/j.psychsport.2006.12.005.

Miedl, S., Peters, J., & Büchel, C. (2012). Altered neural reward representations in pathological gamblers revealed by delay and probability discounting. *Archives of General Psychiatry, 69*, 177–186. https://doi.org/10.1001/archgenpsychiatry.2011.1552.

Montano, D., & Kasprzyk, D. (2015). Theory of unreasoned action, theory of planned behavior and the Intergrated behavioral model. In K. Glanz, B. Rimer, & K. Vizwanath (Eds.), *Health behavior: Theory, research, and practice* (pp. 95–124). San Francisco: Wiley.

Nilsen, H. (2009). Influence on student academic behaviour through motivation, self-efficacy and value expectation: An action research project to improve learning. *Issues in Informing Science and Information Technology, 6*, 545–556.

Parkerson, E., Harris, B., Langdon, J., & Czech, D. (2015). *Using a motivational general-mastery imagery intervention to improve the self-efficacy of youth gymnasts*. Goergia Southern University. Retrieved from https://digitalcommons.georgiasouthern.edu/etd/1257/.

Porcelli, A., & Delgado, H. (2017). Stress and decision making: Effects on valuation, learning, and risk-taking. *Current Opinion in Behavioral Sciences, 14*, 33–39. https://doi.org/10.1016/j.cobeha.2016.11.015.

Poulsen, A., Rodger, S., & Ziviani, J. (2006). Understanding children's motivation from a self-determination theoretical perspective: Implications for practice. *Australian Occupational Therapy Journal, 53*(2), 78–86. https://doi.org/10.1111/j.1440-1630.2006.00569.x.

Robbins, T. (2020). *TOp 20 Most inspiring Tony Robbins quotes*. Retrieved from Goalcast.com: https://www.goalcast.com/2016/08/18/top-20-inspiring-tony-robbins-quotes/.

Stajkovic, A., & Luthans, F. (2003). Social cognitive theory and self efficacy. In L. B. Poter (Ed.), *Motivation and work behavior* (11th ed., pp. 126–140). Boston: McGraw Hill.

Tremblay, M. A., Blanchard, C., Taylor, S., Pelletier, L., & Villeneuve, M. (2009). Work extrinsic and intrinsic motivation scale: Its value for organizational research. *Canadian Journal of Behavioural Science, 41*, 213–226. https://doi.org/10.1037/a0015167.

Tzur, K., Ganzach, Y., & Pazy, A. (2016). On the positive and negative effects of self-efficacy on performance: Reward as a moderator. *Human Performance, 29*(5), 361–377. https://doi.org/10.1080/08959285.2016.1192631.

van de Laar, K., & van de Bijl, J. (2001). Strategies enhancing self-efficacy in diabetis education: A review. *Scholarly Inquiry for Nursing Practice, 15*(13), 235–248.

Vroom, V., Porter, L., & Lawler, E. (2005). Expectancy theories. In J. Miner (Eds.), *Organizational behavior: Essential theories of motivation and leadership* (Vol. 1: Theories of motivation, pp. 94–113). Armonk, NY: M.E. Sharpe.

Wery, J., & Thomson, M. (2013). Motivational strategies to enhance effective learning in teaching struggling students. *Brtish Journal of Learning Support, 28*, 103. https://doi.org/10.1111/1467-9604.12027.

Will, G., Rutledge, R., Moutoussis, M., & Dolan, R. (2017). Neural and computational processes underlying dynamic changes in self-esteem. *eLife, 6*, e28098. https://doi.org/10.7554/eLife.28098.

Wise, J., & Trunnel, E. (2001). The influence of sources of self-efficacy upon efficacy strength. *Journal of Sport and Exercise Psychology, 23*(4), 268–280. https://doi.org/10.1123/jsep.23.4.268.

Zulkosky, K. (2009). Self-efficacy: A concept analysis. *Nursing Forum, 44*(2), 93–102.

Chapter 12
Motivation, Effort, and Neural Network Modeling: Implications

So what is motivation, and how does understanding it from a neural network perspective inform clinical and neuropsychological practice in specific, and social science in general? Before we start discussing the implications of neural network modeling of motivation, it is logical to provide an overview of what motivation is when defined with a neural network framework.

12.1 Defining Motivation

What Is Motivation?

We have seen how motivation is, in part, a cognitive process that propels a person's behavior either toward or away from a particular object, perceived event, or outcome (Zhang, Berridge, Tindell, Smith, & Aldridge, 2009). Using computational modeling that best represents neural network functioning, of these cognitive processes, motivation can be viewed as a subjective, emotion informed modulation of the perceived probabilistic reward value before the reward is received. Therefore, it reflects an organism's state of wanting of a reward that occurs before the outcome is actually achieved (Shuvaev, Tran, Stephenson-Jones, Li, & Koulakov, 2019). We have also seen how, as a result of life course experiences, these reward values are continually being assessed and recalculated as a function of the predication error network.

While these computational models for motivated behavior, which are best fits for reinforcement learning (RL) models, are mostly concerned with the learning aspect of behavior, we have seen that fluctuations in physiological states, such as confidence and anxiety, can also profoundly affect the construct we call motivation (Zhang et al., 2009). Thus, while in the past, motivation has been defined previously

T. Wasserman, L. Wasserman, *Motivation, Effort, and the Neural Network Model*, Neural Network Model: Applications and Implications,
https://doi.org/10.1007/978-3-030-58724-6_12

as the need-based modulation of reward magnitude, we and others, propose an RL approach to understanding how the neural networks operate as regards motivation. This approach considers motivation as an integral part of the complex calculation which leads to goal-directed action.

Finally, it is important to note, that a neural network model looks at the components of a motivated response as, what can be termed, potentials. These potentials exist as automated routines in long-term memory, ready to be drawn to working memory when the proper trigger is supplied. The stored, highly automated potentials exist to be called upon, and are utilized, without the benefit of a cognitive assessment. Rather, these assessments, and the actions upon which they are based, have been calculated so many times that the outcome, in terms of goal selection, is almost predetermined. We say almost because, as we have seen, state-like factors have the potential to alter even the most highly automated motivationally based response. In this form, motivation represents a sort of potential for action that exists before the motor component is activated.

Motivation as a Continuum or Multiple Forms of Motivation?

It hypothetically might be better to label this potential motivation as something different and separate from the motivation that is infused with motor/action components. This is because motivation infused by motoric components represents the latest iteration of the valuation of the various stimuli available for action. The selected action is the most valued at that time. At another time and place it might not be. Therefore, the choice with the highest potential is not always the choice selected.

At first glance it might be attractive to label both activities as motivation because, speculating on two or more different forms of motivation may have value for behavioral descriptions of the activity. In the end, this bifurcation does not match with how we envision the development of higher order cognitive/emotional constructs. We propose that motivation can best be viewed as a uniform, core process that ranges from a potential for certain salient actions to actual attempts to achieve goals and act in accordance with values. Our propensity would be to view it this way as human brains are both efficient and effort saving, and therefore, designing two distinct processes would be neither efficient or effort saving. We think it better to be able to identify a core component to human goal seeking behavior (motivation) that recruits other network components as the task and situation demands. Motoric elements would be added when a particular choice was made to seek a particular desired outcome. These motor requirements further inform and modify the value of the original choice.

Developmentally, this complex behavior would have to emanate from a basic inborn human response or reflex. As we have seen, the inborn fight-or-flight response might is likely the perfect place to start.

The Ever Changing Development of Motivation. The Role of Error Prediction and Value

Motivation is a construct that describes an aspect of the operation of the human learning system that is specifically designed to cause a person to pursue a goal. Anthropologically, these goals were initially, fairly elemental and included the basics necessary for survival, such as food, shelter, and reproduction. Over the course of time they have developed into a complex web of extrinsic, and then intrinsic goals, objectives, and values. To accomplish this task, the basic fight-or-flight reaction has been modified over time by a combination of inborn human temperamental characteristics and life experiences. This modification is in part based on the operation of error prediction network in concert with the reward network to produce a system of ever evolving valuations of goals and objectives. These valuations are never truly fixed. They are constantly being modified and shaped by experience. The error prediction network and learning-related networks work in concert with the limbic system to allow affect laden experiences to inform the process of valuation. These networks, operating in concert, produce a cognitive process we call motivation. Like most networks, the motivation system of networks is recruited when the task demands of the situation require them.

Finally, with sufficient repetition, the valuations created by the above process are stored in working memory in a highly automated way. They represent a state of readiness, to be called upon to propel human goal seeking action. Every time they are called into operation, the results of the behavior they initiate are appraised and the valuation of the goal in question is altered in response. It is important to recognize that even these highly automated potentials cannot perfectly predict motivated behavior. The stored appraisal is still modifiable based on the environmental context in which the person finds themselves when the potential is triggered.

Motivation Is a State and a Trait and Probably Something Else as Well

As we have seen, motivation has both state-like and trait-like properties. It is clear that people are born with specific tolerances of risk aversion, and that these tolerances can be thought of as falling along a continuum from very low to very high. These tolerances are best represented as inborn temperamental characteristics that are then shaped and developed based upon the life course experiences of the individual (Mehregan, Hosseinzadeh, & Emadi, 2018) (Kettlewell, 2018) (Leung, Cloninger, Hong, Cloninger, & Eley, 2019). This shaping of this temperamental predisposition leads to a complex packages of cognitions, arousal, motor, and affectual components that we call motivation. This package of potential responses is stored in memory and available, through highly automated processes, for use when specific stimuli, either intrinsically of extrinsically are encountered. While we have noted that these properties of motivation can rightly lead to the conclusion that certain classes of motivated behavior have very trait-like properties, we have noted that even the most automated of these processes can be influenced by the immediate environmental context. This implies that a person's motivational state is never entirely predictable because circumstances can lead to change in any one particular moment. There is clear research to support the idea that state-like measures of motivation are better predictors of performance than are trait-like measures (Van Iddekinge, Aguinis, Mackey, & DeOrtentiis, 2018). This is specifically an issue in the treatment of disorders of mental health where research clearly indicated the construct of motivation to change is best described as a transient state related to specific, and complex, behavioral changes (Tambling, 2019). These state-like properties fit well with the idea that valuation is constantly being modified based upon current experience and analysis.

There are models to help us understand this particular aspect of motivation. Predictive and reactive control systems (PARCS) theory proposes that people utilize separate neural systems for dealing with different types of environments (Tops, Luu, Boksem, & Tucker, 2013). These reactive control systems are for dealing with unpredictable, unstable, and novel environments. During reactive control, autonomic, homeostatic, and motor control is guided by feedback from stimuli or cues from the environment. By contrast, predictive control systems are for dealing with predictable, familiar, and stable environments. During predictive control, autonomic, homeostatic, and motor control is guided by internally organized model-based predictions and expectancies that are based on people's prior experiences. Suffice it to say there that there are models and research supporting the idea that there are feedback systems in place that are constantly forward predicating motivational value. These systems predict utilizing contextual factors interacting with factors inherent in the current context. Certainly, conceptualizing a multiplicity of related neural networks which share a core group of functions is entirely consistent with neural network modeling. Different task demands require different elements for their solution. The sum of this all, is that no two situations are exactly alike when it comes to predicting motivational value of any particular goal or objective. This is true regardless of whether those values are externally or internally generated and mediated.

Take for example, what happens in the typical approach avoidance conflict. Approach-avoidance conflicts occur when there is one goal or event that has both positive and negative effects or characteristics that make the goal appealing and unappealing simultaneously. A double approach–avoidance conflict is a situation that generates conflict when a person is confronted with two goals or options wherein each has significant attractive and unattractive features. For example, marriage is a momentous decision that has both positive and negative aspects. Working on or leaving a marriage can have its own set of positive and negative variables. Marriage therapy is a highly encountered reason for referral in clinical settings and therapists will attest to the often encountered approach-avoidance sequences the client often goes through in their attempt to both decide and follow through with their chosen course of action. The issue to focus on here is what happens to the value of those positive and negative elements as you move toward selecting one choice or another; they change. Any seasoned clinician can relate to the vacillating that occurs as the therapy process proceeds. As you move farther from a choice, leaving for example, its perceived value (positives) increases and the negatives, staying, decrease. If you turn and move toward the competitor choice, in this case staying, the original choice's positive valuation increases and the negative decreases. The client often vacillates back and forth until they are stuck. The valuation is in flux depending on feedback. In support of this example, research has established that a hierarchical model of approach-avoidance social motivation shows differential predictive patterns for goals depending on context. Again, highly relevant for example, to marital issues. Take for example, the scenario in which someone is contemplating leaving a marriage, but is employed by a company which clearly values marriage as an institution. Herein the implications for a double approach-avoidance conflict become underscored.

12.2 Implications

Now that we know what motivation is and how it is expressed through a neural network system, it is time to take a look at how understanding motivation in this manner would mean for relevant aspects of psychological theory and practice. Motivation is a core element of most form of human behavior. Therefore the implications of understanding motivation from a neural network perspective will be ubiquitous throughout psychological theory and practice.

When we started on this book we recognized that reformulating how motivation was thought about as a process would impact many areas of both psychological and neuropsychological practice. We were not disappointed. Understanding how motivation is functionalized by neural networks offers significant insight, but at the same time provides sharp limitations to extrapolated assumptions related to motivation psychologically and neuropsychologically. So it's about time that we looked at some of these implications in detail.

Effort Testing

There are implications for effort testing in neuropsychology. There are essential questions that neuropsychologists are always concerned about (Kimbell & Maccow, 2011):

- The accuracy of the test data depends on the cooperation and effort of the test taker.
- What if test takers do not perform to the best of their ability and what if effort is less than optimal for the tasks?

There is a growing body of evidence demonstrating significant variability in test-taking motivation for the same individuals at different times of the day between different school classes (Knekta, 2017). This particular study was interesting in that it also highlighted the state-like characteristics of motivation. Knekta found differences in test-taking motivation between school classes, using authentic tests that had different perceived stakes for the same group of pupils. They concluded that test-taking motivation varies between and within tests with different stakes, and that test-taking motivation seems to be one factor affecting test performance. They interpreted the results based on the expectancy-value theory of achievement motivation which understands student motivation as expressed as performance, persistence, and task choice. In this model motivation depends on expectations for success and the value placed on the task. As we have seen this model is well explained within a probabilistic valuation model. Other studies have found similar results (Swerdzewski, Harmes, & Finney, 2011) resulting in recommendations for consideration of embedded effort testing across all tests administered in a session.

As pertains to effort, based on the above, while it seems accurate to say that repeat effort testing can assess general motivation predisposition (the trait like qualities of an individual's motivational temperament), you can never be entirely sure that a person is acting in a motivated fashion in the moment. They could have passed an effort probe 10 min prior, but may now be tired, or hungry, or bored, or have to use the bathroom and decide to rush through whatever measure they are taking at the moment. It could mean none of those things. It could just mean that the individual did not like the type of skill being assessed. It could reflect self-image in that they do not believe themselves very competent in this area. Environmental, state, or whatever the issue, while you can have a higher confidence level in a person's general state at the time of assessment using effort indicators (Larrabee, 2012), you can't be 100% sure of the person's level of effort at any given specific time. This is because as it turns out, state and trait dispositions may in fact be present within the response to the same task (Dornyei & Ta Tseng, 2019). They report data that shows that it is reasonable to assume a circular process of motivational task processing in which appropriate signals from the appraisal system concerning a specific task execution trigger needs to activate relevant action control strategies, which in turn further facilitate the execution process. In other words, every action is appraised in its current context and no two contexts are ever the same. The sole exception to this idea occurs when the person fails an effort probe. Then you can be sure that they weren't trying.

Position statements from the National Academy of Neuropsychology and the American Academy of Clinical Neuropsychology (AACN) have recommended routine validity testing in neuropsychological evaluations. The above however, may argue for embedded measures of motivation by task. That is, it may be better to assess motivation for the task itself. There have been efforts in this regard (Sugarman & Axelrod, 2015) using for example, verbal fluency measures, and performance measures such as coding to provide multiple measures of Symptom Validity Tests (SVTs). This would address many issues; however, it may not address for example, outlier scores, which many a clinician has seen being used as the basis of a diagnosis or (learning) disability.

Effort, Error Prediction, Reward, and Mental Health

As is consistent with neural network modeling, processes associated with one set of functions are also recruited in solving other tasks as well. It is easy then, to extrapolate that disruptions of these processes are implicated in behaviors associated with mental health issues. There is research that demonstrates that this is in fact the case. For example, accurately recognizing and correcting for errors that one has committed would appear to be crucial for strategic behavioral and neuronal adjustments to avoid similar errors in the future. Without correcting for errors, people would engage in the same poorly adaptive behaviors over and over again, or, at the extreme, not survive. In addition, accurately assessing how much your perception of the possibility of success differed from the actual result would be important in determining whether the same response would be repeated. Studies have demonstrated that error awareness and lack of insight related to the impact of behavior on the environment are present in a number of disorders including schizophrenia, attention-deficit hyperactivity disorder (ADHD), and autism spectrum disorders (ASD). In all these disorders, the performance of the monitoring and assessment system is reported as impaired, thereby implicating the error recognition network (Klein, Ullsperger, & Danielmeier, 2013). Individuals with obsessive-compulsive disorder (OCD) have been found to show exaggerated error responses and prediction error learning signals in a variety of EEG and fMRI tasks, with data converging on the anterior cingulate cortex as a key locus of dysfunction (Murray et al., 2019). Thus, it may be entirely possible that we have had this backward. That is, ADHD or OCD per se, may not be the cause of error prediction inaccuracy, but rather, error prediction inaccuracy or disruption may in some way cause some of the behaviors that comprise ADHD and OCD.

Also taken into account must be the insula, a brain region that appears consistently involved in error awareness processing research. The insular has been implicated in both error awareness and, with anterior insular regions, being involved in conscious error processing. Klein et al. (2013) argue that the insular cortex, because of its cytoarchitectonic layout, and its functional and structural connectivity, is perfectly suited to play a vital role in error awareness. The insula, with its role of processing interoceptive information, might be relaying information between networks which is involved in external attention and supports error awareness. They note that while likely a gradient, impaired information relay can result in deficient to profound problems.

Failure to accurately assess perceptual error can also lead to behavior that is integrally involved with certain disorders for mental health. Klein et al. (2013), in their review article point out that volume reduction of the insular cortex in schizophrenia has been shown multiple times and damage to the insula could under lie the sensory integration deficits common to schizophrenia. They go on to highlight studies associated with error awareness and performance errors in ADHD and autism. There is also research that people with eating disorders, particularly Anorexia Nervosa, have poor cognitive flexibility (Tchanturia et al., 2011). This leads to repetitive behavior due to failure to shift set. Poor cognitive flexibility has been demonstrated to be related to, in part, failure to accurately change error prediction based on experience (Hauser, Iannaccone, Walitza, Brandeis, & Bremae, 2015). Thus the rigidity and poor body image demonstrated in eating disorders may be due in large part to the deficient operation of the error prediction system. By extension poor modulation of the error prediction system may be related to things such as obsessive-compulsive disorder as well.

It is possible that developmentally maladaptive changes to the operation of the error recognition system may be related to the emergence of adult disorders of mental health.

As we have seen, multiple dopaminergic neurocognitive systems contribute simultaneously to reinforcement learning by incrementally updating the value of choices, while the prefrontal cortex contributes different computations, such as actively maintaining precise information in working memory. What happens when this system goes awry? There is research to suggest that the development of reinforcement learning processes plays a protracted role in changes in learning during adolescent development. This occurs when working memory is overloaded and compensated by reinforcement learning processes in the brain. Both of these processes are interfaced with executive skills. Late adolescent maturation is widely associated with the development of higher cognitive resources, including adult-like working memory (and the use of increasingly complex learning strategies. The development of these forms of higher cognition are most often attributed to the development of prefrontal cortex, which does not reach functional or structural maturation until late in the second decade or even middle of the third decade of life (Master et al., 2020). Therefore one could speculate that error-related disruptions of this system in late adolescence are responsible for the appearance of disorders.

Adolescence is known to be a period of increasing incidence of several classes of psychiatric illnesses, including anxiety and mood disorders, psychosis, eating disorders, personality disorders, and substance abuse. The pathophysiology of these disorders is being increasingly understood as arising from aberrations of maturational changes that normally occur in the adolescent brain (Giedd, Keshavan, & Paus, 2008). They note that adolescence is characterized by major changes in the neural networks that subserve higher cognitive functions, reasoning and interpersonal interactions, cognitive control of emotions, risk-vs-reward appraisal and motivation. They conclude by stating "Not surprisingly, when not adequately surmounted, it is precisely these challenges that increase the risk of cognitive, affective and addictive disorders."(p. 960). It is easy to see how increasingly inaccurate error modifications could contribute to this process. For example, they point out that "the abnormal engagement of brain regions to emotional facial expressions in adolescents may underlie realistic appraisal of emotions and thereby predispose to anxiety and depression."

Child psychology practices are full of children who are referred for not performing successfully in school. Often these children are themselves frustrated, indicating that in their own perceptions they "did try." Parents or teachers often respond that they need to "try harder." But isn't it possible that they did put forth effort, but miscalculated the amount of effort necessary.

As we have seen, people tend to use the level of effort necessary to solve a task and rarely expend more effort than necessary. Neuropsychology reports often speak to "effort." Statements like "John appeared to work to the best of his ability" are likely, but just likely questionable and not at all accurate. If an examinee did do well, the best that we can probably ascribe is that "John consistently put forth the effort required to solve the problems presented to him."

This second statement brings forth the possibility of a number of interesting scenarios. For example, suppose that John did poorly on the test. Is this an example of a young man who is putting forth poor effort secondary to a paucity of motivation, or a young man who consistently fails to accurately gauge the effort required to successfully complete the task, or has poor error awareness.

The next possible scenario is also of great importance. It speaks to the current diagnostic system and what the current authors perceive as an inherent flaw in nosology. Specifically, in most instances these young people have their diminished performance ascribed to a lack of motivation which is in turn ascribed to a disorder of mental health (ADHD, OCD, Depression, etc.). What if that wasn't at all the reason? What if John's error prediction system is off, and the assessments he is making are inaccurate as a result. There might not be a need to conceptualize further. That is, the idea that every human is born with a perfectly functional error prediction system seems a bit farfetched. We have discussed how the current mental health nosology encourages researchers to miss this point. In fact, the current nosology dictates that if one has a disorder of motivation, effort is reduced to a secondary characteristic of a primary mental health disorder such as ADHD. We have argued for consideration of a group of motivational disorders in their own right as, speaking to this point, not every child with a diagnosis of ADHD has poor motivation, nor does every child with impacted motivation have ADHD.

We go into detail here, not to thoroughly explore the operation of the error prediction and modulation system in the role of mental health. We do so in order to point out how the brain recruits the network components for multiple tasks in a manner that is predicted by computational neural network modeling. While it would, we suppose, be accurate to state that motivation plays a prominent role in many psychiatric disorders it is probably more accurate to say that error prediction lies at the core of problems in both these associated areas. That's why when you see problems in one area, you are much more likely to see the other.

A Word to Therapists

We have worked extensively on trying to incorporate this work into our clinical practice (Wasserman & Wasserman, 2017). We have found that helping clients frame their discussion of motivation and effort according to these principles is quite helpful. We structure the discussion by breaking down motivation into three general steps.

1. We tend to pursue what we like the best.
2. We pursue what we believe we are willing to make an effort to get.
3. We only will try if we believe our effort will be successful.

Most clients can see where they have problems. For example, many of our unmotivated people believe that they will fail no matter what effort they make. If they believe that, it doesn't matter how much they want it or how much they are willing to try. Take for example, Gina, a 26-year-old women in treatment for depression associated with poor arousal and lack of socialization. After some discussion, Gina said that she was unwilling to try therapy suggestions to practice the socialization skills that she was taught. Based on her history, she was convinced that she would fail to use them properly. In fact, observations of Gina's interactions with others in the office suite highlighted very poor self-awareness including avoidance of face-to-face contact, averting and a lack of responding to social greetings. Gina was also convinced that people would see how painfully shy she was and decide that she wasn't worth the effort. No matter how much therapy she had, or how many times she practiced in the office, these two beliefs prevented her from trying on her own. Highlighting and making the above three ideas explicit allowed Gina to tackle them head on, and she agreed to a very controlled trial at which she was very successful. Even then she insisted that the success was an exception. It took several practice sessions to overcome and alter these cognitions. Changing her prediction of failure was the key to therapeutic progress. There are several other characteristics of motivation, viewed through a neural network lens that will also impact Gina's treatment. Let's take a look at a couple of these.

Motivation Improves Through Behavioral Mastery and Analysis of Errors

As a result of her desire to be perfect, and avoid making errors, Gina was missing an essential element of the motivational process. This essential component of the motivational process is the analysis of errors related to attempts at goal attainment. This analysis leads a person to either increase or decrease their expectations of future success based upon actual experience. These expectations are always being recalculated based upon experience. Without this error analysis expectation does not change and, subsequently the motivated behavior that derives from unchanging assessment would also not change. As a result of her anxiety, Gina had eliminated this activity from her daily behavior. It is quite logical to assume that actual improvement in terms of motivational power would only occur if these assessments were actually created as a result of actual attempts but were also altered to reflect an increasing likelihood of success. The best way to insure that this occurs is to actually engage in goal seeking behavior and demonstrate mastery by having the behavior be successful in obtaining the goal. If that happens, the expectations of success are favorably altered, and the resulting power of motivation related to that goal is improved. If that doesn't happen, or if the person is unsuccessful, the resulting feed forward expectation of future success would diminish. In other words, motivation would decrease. This implies that to improve motivation it is necessary to engage in successful behavioral practice. Without error analysis of actual behavioral action, sustainable improvement in motivation should not be expected.

Therein in lies the secret to improving motivated behavior toward those goals and objectives that are important for society at large, but not among a specific person's priorities. Motivation is improved if the effort required to reach a goal is considered by a person to be reasonable. It also improves if the person has a high expectation that the behavior required to reach the goal will pay off. Mastery elevates both of these factors Mastery decreases the cognitive effort required to reach a goal, and mastery proves to the person that they have the requisite abilities to be successful. Mastery therefore directly impacts expected valuation with the result being that the particular goal or objective will be more highly valued in the future.

The necessity for behavioral action and related mastery to be included in a program of change has been demonstrated in a number of settings including school leadership (Holmes & Parker, 2018), student instruction (Forsyth & Archer, 1997), weight loss intervention (Barnes & Cassidy, 2018), psychotherapy (Tambling, 2019), and safety programming (Geller & Geller, 2019) to name but a few.

Motivation in Therapy Is Facilitated by Behavioral Action and Mastery

There is significant research pointing to the fact that motivation and motivation informed therapy is an essential element of psychotherapy (Wastermann, Grosse Holtforth, & Michalak, 2017). Therapists are always working to motivate clients to try more adaptive solutions for their behavior and emotional difficulties. This idea plays an important role in Gina's treatment as Gina was refusing to act at all. If this idea is correct, as we believe it is, Gina was not going to make any movement in therapy until this situation was corrected.

We have spoken about research that indicates that a major element of most psychotherapy, verbal persuasion, by itself is not very effective in encouraging a person to make behavioral change (Bandura, 1977). That is not to say that verbal persuasion does not work at all. There is clear evidence that, as part of a package of interventions, verbal persuasion can be effective in producing change (Pica & Howell, 2018). The self-efficacy model says that people improve their self-efficacy, which is defined in a belief that they can control the processes leading to an outcome, though the operation of five related/interactive processes: exerting control over inner processes of goal setting, self-monitoring, feedback, problem solving, and self-evaluation. As we have seen these cognitive processes are verbally based in therapy and essential in preparing the belief systems that would lead a person to predict that they would be successful in an attempt to obtain a goal. From a neural network perspective these processes looks remarkably similar to the mastery, feedback, and error analysis functions performed by neural networks. That is as it should be because these constructs described in self-efficacy theory merely represent behavioral descriptions of the operation of the neural network.

All of this leads to the conclusion that predictions are not sufficient to cause behavior change on their own. Neither is encouragement or the uncovering of long automated emotional or behavioral routines. While these might be important precursors or contributors to the change process, the one inescapable fact is that they must be accompanied by behavioral practice to cause the client to choose the new, more adaptive, behaviors in the future. The new behaviors must be practiced until they are automated. Automation reduces the necessity of cognitive effort. It also leads to improved mastery (Wasserman & Wasserman, 2017). Both are essential for improved motivation to select the new, more adaptive sets of behaviors that are required for therapeutic change. In neural network terms, the person's estimate of the probability of success would improve. This estimate of improvement is one way to understand the motivational value of the stimulus, object, or goal.

We have seen how neural network modeling has significant implications for much of what psychologists and neuropsychologists do. These implications should encourage us to take a closer look at our current practices and perhaps change them to reflect our improved understanding. Two major underlying points, that all therapy should include behavioral practice and mastery work and secondly that one can never totally know whether a client is performing at their maximum on psychological tests have profound implications for current practice.

Personality Models That Include Neural Network Modeling of Motivation

We are not alone in trying to understand how motivation can be understood in terms of the actions of specific neural networks operating interdependently. There have been other attempts to formulate neural network models of motivation. We suspect there will be many more. Looking at another attempt might be informative. Read et al. (2010), using an algorithm model, provide a model of personality that is driven by two general levels of motivation, with an additional general control system that operates on the motivational systems. They describe two general motivational systems, which have been variously termed approach and avoidance systems: behavioral approach systems (BAS) and behavioral inhibition systems (BIS). The approach system governs response to rewarding stimuli and strongly parallels the broad trait of extraversion, whereas the avoidance system governs response to punishment and aversive stimuli and strongly parallels the broad trait of neuroticism, particularly its facets of anxiety and fearfulness. Each of these two broad motivational systems subsumes and moderates a set of more specific motives, such as affiliation, sex, dominance, avoiding social rejection, and avoiding physical harm. The behavior of specific motives is a joint function of characteristics of the broad motivational system of which it is a part and of its own specific parameters. Moderating the activity of these motivational systems is a general "control system," characterized as a disinhibition and constraint system. The inhibitory processes of this control system moderate the activity of the motivational systems and related behavior.

In addition to the critical role played by these motivational systems and by the general inhibitory process (disinhibition and constraint), the model has two other essential components. One component provides for a representation of the situations to which the individual is responding. They propose that situations are modeled by a feature layer, which represents salient or motive-relevant attributes of the situation. A second component represents the resources that an individual possesses (e.g., intellect, flexibility) that are important in the pursuit and attainment of the individual's goals. These resources are thought of as key components of traits. They are modeled by a resource layer, which represents the presence or absence of various motive-relevant resources that the individual directly possesses as part of their person. There are other kinds of resources that comprise situationally driven elements of the environment which are modeled in the feature layer.

The purpose of the model is to demonstrate how motivation impacts the operation of personality. To the current authors, this is a model clearly based on neuroscience research, from an evolutionary perspective which is utilizing the basic fight-or-flight reflex as its basis, which leads to approach avoidance, which supports the life course perspective of how personality and motivation continually impact each other across the life span, with an emphasis on the constant interplay between reward valuation and personality, beginning at the beginning of the life of the organism. It adds dimension in helping us flesh out the differences which arise in individuals as they create a unique personality.

What About Those Other Theories of Motivation?

We want to state in the strongest possible terms that discussing the neural network underpinnings of motivation in no way supplants what has come before in terms of other theories of motivation contributing to the operation of human behavior. These theories do an amazing job at describing what motivated behavior looks like after it is created. We hope you agree with us that our work is additive and enriching. What we have done is describe how the complex patterns of behavior, emotion, and cognition are processed in the human brain and are integrated to produce complicated goal seeking behavior. As we have endeavored to point out, much of what has come before has consisted of descriptions of types of motivated behavior and thought that were, for the most part, informed by description and categorization of those behaviors and thoughts. These models tell us how motivation looks when humans do it and often suggest what things may trigger such behavior. These triggers at the fundamental level may consist of basic survival things such as food and water. At their most developed, they can be quite esoteric, such as self-actualization.

By understanding how constructs such as self-actualization play out across the human connectome we can better conjecture how these concepts develop and be more effective in designing developmental experiences that support its development. The idea here is not to develop a reductionist model that dismisses all of the marvelous things that the human brain can create. The idea here is to understand how the brain does what it does and to understand the strengths and weaknesses inherent in its operation. By building upon basic skills and continuously integrating new network problem solving activities the human brain is capable of incredible things. All we wanted to do is tell you how we think it does that.

References

Bandura, A. (1977). Self-efficacy: Toward a unifying theory of behavioral change. *Psychological Review, 84*(2), 191–215.

Barnes, M., & Cassidy, T. (2018). Diet, exercise and motivation in weight reduction: The role of psychological capital and stress: Diet, exercise and motivation in weight reduction. *Journal of Nursing and Health Care, 9*(5), 555775. https://doi.org/10.19080/JOJNHC.2018.09.555775.

Dornyei, Z., & Ta Tseng, W. (2019). Motivational processing in interactional tasks. In Z. Wen & M. Ahmadian (Eds.), *Researching L2 task performance and pedagogy: In honour of Peter Skehan* (pp. 55–66). Amsterdam: John Benjamin Publishing.

Forsyth, D., & Archer, C. (1997). Technologically assisted instruction and student mastery, motivation, and matriculation. *Teaching of Psychology, 24*(3), 155–159. https://doi.org/10.1207/s15328023top2403_17.

Geller, E., & Geller, K. (2019). *Psychological science for safety success, Part 3 how to inspire self-motivation & empowerment.* PSJ PROFESSIONAL SAFETY. Retrieved from https://search.proquest.com/openview/2ef2232a56a27472bd1fd726c035c935/1?pq-origsite=gscholar&cbl=47267.

Giedd, J., Keshavan, M., & Paus, T. (2008). Why do many psychiatric disorders emerge during adolescence? *Nature Reviews. Neuroscience, 9*(12), 947–957. https://doi.org/10.1038/nrn2513.

Hauser, T., Iannaccone, R., Walitza, S., Brandeis, S., & Bremae, S. (2015). Cognitive flexibility in adolescence: Neural and behavioral mechanisms of reward prediction error processing in adaptive decision making during development. *NeuroImage, 104*(1), 347–354. https://doi.org/10.1016/j.neuroimage.2014.09.018.

Holmes, W., & Parker, M. (2018). The relationship between behavioural integrity, competence, goodwill, trustworthiness, and motivating language of a principal. *School Leadership & Management, 38*(4), 435–456. https://doi.org/10.1080/13632434.2018.1430687.

Kettlewell, N. (2018). *Risk preference dynamics around life events.* The University of Sydney: Economics Working Paper Series. Retrieved from http://econ-wpseries.com/2018/201807.pdf.

Kimbell, A., & Maccow, G. (2011). *Assessment of suboptimal effort.* Pearson. Retrieved from https://images.pearsonclinical.com/images/PDF/webinar/Suboptimal-Effort-Webinar-Handout.pdf.

Klein, T. M., Ullsperger, M., & Danielmeier, C. (2013). Error awareness and the insula: Links to neurological and psychiatric diseases. *Frontiers in Human Neuroschience, 7*, 14. https://doi.org/10.3389/fnhum.2013.00014.

Knekta, E. (2017). Are all pupils equally motivated to do their best on all tests? Differences in reported test-taking motivation within and between tests with different stakes. *Scandinavian Journal of Educational Research, 61*(1), 95–111. https://doi.org/10.1080/00313831.2015.1119723.

Larrabee, G. (2012). Performance validity and symptom validity in neuropsychological assessment. *Journal of the International Neuropsychological Society, 18*, 625–631. https://doi.org/10.1017/S1355617712000240.

Leung, J., Cloninger, C., Hong, B., Cloninger, K., & Eley, D. (2019). Temperament and character profiles of medical students associated with tolerance of ambiguity and perfectionism. *Brain and Cognition PeerJ, 7*, e7109. https://doi.org/10.7717/peerj.7109.

Master, S., Eckstein, M., Gotlieb, N., Dahl, R., Wilbrecht, L., & Collins, L. (2020). Distentangling the systems contributing to changes in learning during adolescence. *Developmental Cognitive Neuroscience, 41*, 100732. https://doi.org/10.1016/j.dcn.2019.100732.

Mehregan, M., Hosseinzadeh, M., & Emadi, M. (2018). The mediating role of affect in the relationship between the big five factor personality and risk aversion: A structural model. *International Journal of Applied Behavioral Sciences (IJABS), 5*(2), 28–36.

Murray, G., Knolle, F., Ersche, K., Craig, K., Abbott, S., Shaila, S., et al. (2019). Dopaminergic drug treatment remediates exaggerated cingulate prediction error responses in obsessive-compulsive disorder. *Psychopharmacology, 236*, 2325–2336. https://doi.org/10.1007/s00213-019-05292-2.

Pica, K., & Howell, D. (2018). A model to increase rehabilitation adherence to home exercise. *Musculoskeletal Care, 16*, 233–237. https://doi.org/10.1002/msc.1194.

Read, S., Monroe, B., Brownstein, A., Yang, Y., Chopra, G., & Miller, L. (2010). A neural network model of the structure and dynamics of human personality. *Psychological Review, 117*(1), 61–92. https://doi.org/10.1037/a0018131.

Shuvaev, S., Tran, N., Stephenson-Jones, M., Li, B., & Koulakov, A. (2019). *Neural networks with motivation.* Retrieved from arxiv.org: https://arxiv.org/pdf/1906.09528.pdf.

Sugarman, M., & Axelrod, B. (2015). Embedded measures of performance validity using verbal fluency tests in a clinical sample. *Applied Neuropsychology: Adult, 22*, 141–146. https://doi.org/10.1080/23279095.2013.873439.

Swerdzewski, P. J., Harmes, J. C., & Finney, S. J. (2011). Two approaches for identifying low-motivated students in a low-stakes assessment context. *Applied Measurement in Education, 24*(2), 162–168. https://doi.org/10.1080/08957347.2011.555217.

Tambling, R. (2019). A critical evaluation of motivation to change conceptualization, measurement, and utility in counseling and psychotherapy. *The Family Journal, 23*, 106648071983339. https://doi.org/10.1177/1066480719833399.

Tchanturia, K., Harrison, A., Davies, H., Roberts, M., Oldershaw, A., Nakazato, M., et al. (2011). Cognitive flexibility and clinical severity in eating disorders. *PLoS One, 6*(6), e20462. https://doi.org/10.1371/journal.pone.0020462.

Tops, M., Luu, P., Boksem, M., & Tucker, D. (2013). The roles of reactive and prospective behavioral/physiological programs in resilience. In M. Kent, M. Davis, & J. Reich (Eds.), *The resilience handbook: Approaches to stress and trauma* (pp. 15–32). London: Routledge.

Van Iddekinge, C., Aguinis, H., Mackey, J., & DeOrtentiis, P. (2018). A meta-analysis of the interactive, additive, and relative effects of cognitive ability and motivation on performance. *Journel of Managment, 44*(1), 249–279. https://doi.org/10.1177/0149206317702220.

Wasserman, T., & Wasserman, L. (2017). *Neurocognitive learning therapy: Theory and practice.* New York: Springer.

Wastermann, S., Grosse Holtforth, M., & Michalak, J. (2017). Motivation in psychotherapy. In R. Ryan (Ed.), *The Oxford handbook of human motivation* (pp. 417–441). New York: Oxford University Press.

Zhang, J., Berridge, K., Tindell, A., Smith, K., & Aldridge, J. (2009). A neural computational model of incentive salience. *PLoS Computational Biology, 5*(7), e1000437. https://doi.org/10.1371/journal.pcbi.1000437.

Index

T. Wasserman, L. Wasserman, *Motivation, Effort, and the Neural Network Model*, Neural Network Model: Applications and Implications,
https://doi.org/10.1007/978-3-030-58724-6

The manufacturer's authorised representative in the EU is Springer
Nature Customer Service Centre GmbH, Europaplatz 3, 69115 Heidelberg,
Germany. If you have any concerns regarding our products, please
contact ProductSafety@springernature.com

Printed and bound by CPI Group (UK) Ltd, Croydon, CR0 4YY
30/09/2026
02225465-0017